Metabolic Stimulation System

– DAVE SHEAHAN –

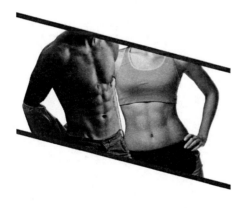

Printed and bound in England by www.printondemand-worldwide.com

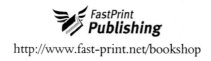

http://www.fast-print.net/bookshop

METABOLIC STIMULATION SYSTEM
Copyright © Dave Sheahan 2017

The right of Dave Sheehan to be identified as the author of this work has been asserted by him in accordance with the Copyright, Designs and Patents Act 1988 and any subsequent amendments thereto.

A catalogue record for this book is available from the British Library

ISBN 978-178456-450-6

First published 2017 by
FASTPRINT PUBLISHING
Peterborough, England.

Table Of Contents

Preface

In 2010 I published my last book "6 Weeks To A Cover Model Body". Since then people from all over the world just like you have transformed not just their bodies but their lives in just weeks by following the programme. My 6 Week CMB Bootcamp business and Home Workout System were born out of this book and it has been truly amazing playing a role in thousands of lives being transformed during the last 6 years. A Mind/Body/Health Transformation impacts much more than just your confidence and self esteem. It positively impacts your entire life which you are going to experience during your Metabolic Stimulation System journey which starts now! You have taken the crucial first step by investing in this book. My "6 Weeks To A Cover Model Body" book was the result of dedicating 15 years to researching and testing the most up to date scientific body transformation strategies. I am someone who believes in the Kaizen method of learning – constant and never ending. Therefore I have never stopped researching, learning and experimenting and I never will.

I was excited to write Metabolic Stimulation System armed with 6 further years of knowledge and results. My MSS principles and step by step programme will now see you achieve even faster lifelong results by implementing what I have learned since 2010. I am now armed with new strategies as well as variations on those in my previous book. Some of what I am going to share in MSS will be a total 360 on what I shared previously. Hence why this book you hold in your hands is such a powerful and impactful follow up to my previous book. I am so excited to finally have this book written and now in your hands. The hundreds of clients who I have coached using this programme over the last 6 years have experienced incredible results. I am truly excited for you.

You would expect that at a time with so much information available and so many "experts" that there would be less confusion. You would expect that it would now be clear as to what works to achieve not just fast but lifelong results that will also easily be maintained. However the opposite is true. Now more so than ever. There is more confusion now than there was 5 or 10 years ago. The internet, a blessing in so many ways, has just become a major source of confusion and conflicting opinions on what is effective. There are now so many "experts" who are basically robbing your hard earned money with ineffective diets and programmes hyped up and brought into your consciousness by heavy investment in marketing. More weightloss and body transformation books are being published than ever before. There are now so many websites, blogs, youtube channels, ebooks, webinars and much more. But sadly, much to my frustration as an observer, all this available information is just worsening the situation. Confusion reigns. What makes me most mad is that this is a time when more people than ever are crying out for a real solution and are prepared and ready to follow a step by step plan.

I want to pose a question. When you look at the weightloss industry does it really want you to get in shape and easily maintain it? Of course not. Confusion is great for the industry. It allows it to keep churning out new potions, pills, detoxes, gimmicks and programmes. And even when you look at "experts" how many of them truly give you all the steps you need to both achieve and maintain results? Not many. Don't get me wrong there are some in the industry I highly respect and admire but there are far more that are spouting a load of crap, pretending to be experts and fooling people into investing in them. Like with the pharmaceutical industry there is no profit in healthy happy people. And both the industry and certain experts want you to continuously invest in them versus giving you the step by step solution. This way you are just kept in the same cycle of trying to get in shape while being bombarded by shake diets, detox plans, revolutionary systems etc. And this really drives me mad. Don't get me wrong I love having people like you investing in everything I bring out. But I know that what I release will always be quality and even with this book you have everything you need to achieve fast lifelong results.

The widespread confusion and how the industry is run are the 2 main reasons why I decided to write Metabolic Stimulation System. I also wanted to share all the new strategies I now know which my global clients implement daily for even faster results than on my programmes years ago. I set out on this book project with a determination to ensure that it would be (which it is in my opinion) the most comprehensive step by step programme for not just successful body transformation but most importantly for lifestyle change. MSS is focused on guiding you step by step in regaining control of your mind/body/health and in a way that is easily maintained for life without any deprivation or negative association with exercise. Sound good?

I am passionate about, and dedicated to, giving you all the tools and strategies you need. MSS will allow you to experience your own body transformation in the fastest time and far more importantly in a way that ensures easy maintenance. Lifelong lifestyle change is what our goal is as you read MSS. It is not just a focus on getting in shape for the beach or a wedding or a holiday. Be clear MSS is a fast solution but also a lifelong solution – make sense? Ready to do this?

I am excited for you and I wish I held this book in my hands at the age of 17 when I desperately needed to get in shape and experience all the amazing benefits of doing so.

Are you excited?

Next I will share my personal story and journey in transforming my body and regaining control of my mind/body/health and how becoming a Body For Life Champion changed my life forever. I hope my personal journey inspires you and that you will be able to relate to some or all of it. After the introduction we will go deep into the foundations of my Metabolic Stimulation System. You will be educated on everything you need to know about the 4 key areas for regaining control of your mind/body/health – mindset, exercise, nutrition and sleep. Each one is equally important and a lack of focus on one dramatically decreases your level of success overall. Once I am done teaching you everything you need to know about these 4 areas I will walk you through step by step the Metabolic Stimulation System programme.

This is the solution you have been waiting for. This will be the last programme you will ever need to follow. Are you ready to transform your mind/body/health forever? And to learn how to easily maintain this new body and lifestyle?

Just do yourself and me a big favour!!

Follow through on applying and following the MSS Programme.

I don´t want this book gathering dust on a shelf.

Make a promise to yourself right this moment that you will follow through.

Deal??

Let's go!

Introduction

Dear Reader

When you look in the mirror do you dislike or even feel disgust at what looks back at you? Maybe you even avoid mirrors for this reason? When clients tell me they feel this way it is so sad and I don't say this in a disrespectful way. I mean that nobody should ever experience this. No one should feel so bad about themselves that they avoid looking in mirrors or going clothes shopping or avoid social interactions. You should love yourself, both on the inside and outside. When you truly love yourself you feel complete and attract great things into your life. You are able to make a big difference in the world and to those around you. However when you don't love yourself everything is negatively impacted. When one is in this position they must dig deep and find the strength and will within themselves to take action in starting the journey to change. This is why you should feel proud of yourself holding this book as you have taken that first step to changing everything, not just your body shape. I want to stress this point, and likely will do many times between now and the final page. Another important point I want to stress to you is that knowledge is not power but the implementation of knowledge is. So right this moment make a promise to yourself that you are going to follow and implement all that you learn in this book. You are going to take action on all the steps. When you do I can promise you, hand on heart, that this will be the last time that you will need to take part on such a journey to a positive mindset, a better body, optimal health and most important of all to loving yourself.

Does a stubborn layer of fat remain on your midsection? Seemingly unshiftable despite a lot of sweat, pain and sacrifice? It remains despite all of the energy and time that you have put in? It remains despite much financial investment in gym memberships, personal trainers, bootcamps, exercise classes, weight management programmes, diets, detox plans, pills, shakes, online programmes, home workout dvds and anything else you have followed diligently but without the outcome you desperately wanted to achieve.

Are you sick and tired of putting so much time and effort into shopping, planning, preparing and eating while following what you have been promised is the best fat burning nutrition programme or diet around? Are you fed up of feeling deprived on your current nutrition plan/diet? Are you sick of eating foods you are not particularly fond of and feeling deprived being unable to eat foods that you like? Are you fed up of feeling hungry all the time? Or sick and low on energy as you will on particular diets?

I expect you answered a resounding Yes to most or likely all of the above questions. I have good news for you. The Metabolic Stimulation System will not have you enduring any of these negative experiences and feelings. MSS is the solution you have been searching for. I know you have heard this a million times before.

However this time will be different. Why? Because this book is truly the most comprehensive step by step plan you will ever read which focuses not just on sharing with you what to do but educates you in detail about why you should do it. This way you can fully understand each part of the system and this makes implementation much easier, consistent and likely. When MSS is followed step by step you will experience not just an incredible body transformation but more importantly a positive mind/body/health impact. Your psychology and habits will change forever. This will be experienced within just weeks. Your lifestyle change will be incredible and will be easily maintained forever. We have all followed plans that yielded short term results which then frustratingly reversed within weeks often resulting in being worse off than you were originally. Have you been there before?

Do my promises about Metabolic Stimulation System sound too good to be true? I wouldn't blame you if you thought this way. If I was in your shoes I would feel the same having been repeatedly lied to and misinformed by so many "Experts" of the weightloss industry. I would feel frustrated too if every time I invested in a solution it only gave me some of the formula. I can totally empathise with you and feel your pain and frustration having spent many years of my life busting my ass exercising and rigidly following strict "healthy" nutrition plans and all for minimal improvements. I expect you to be sceptical and you should be. You work hard for your money and your time is the most valuable asset you have so I want you to invest both your money and time wisely with a huge ROI. What I can promise, hand on heart, is that your experience with this book and programme will be different and that my MSS is the real deal. You will experience the proof both while reading this book and then over the next 6 weeks and beyond following the MSS programme. I am looking forward to proving myself right.

My personal frustration and confusion at a lack of results are what motivated me over 20 years ago to research far and wide to find effective body transformation strategies. Also at that time I committed to never relenting on this thirst for knowledge. I made that commitment to myself at that time as I had just taken my first steps towards a career in the fitness industry and was determined to become #1. Many years of indepth research as well as using my body as a guinea pig are what lead to one of my proudest accomplishments – becoming a Body For Life Challenge Champion in 2004. It was Bill Phillips and his BFL programme which was one of my early inspirations and education resources in learning the truth about effective body transformation strategies. Since 2004 I have coached thousands of individuals, just like you, all over the world, in successfully transforming their bodies in just weeks. But the most important result was that most of these people created healthy active lifestyles in the process and with my strategies were able to easily maintain their new bodies. In some cases my clients continued to improve their body shape further dropping more bodyfat and gaining more lean muscle. Some of my clients used their success to become personal trainers and they now inspire others to achieve what they did. They are now changing lives by sharing their journey and the steps involved. Whether you intend to or not you will inspire others to take action as they witness your transformation happening before them. Just wait. There is no greater satisfaction than having a positive impact on other people's lives.

My biggest motivation in writing Metabolic Stimulation System was to make available a comprehensive step by step plan for both fast and lifelong success. I grew frustrated at the widespread confusion despite more information being available than ever before via the internet. I grew frustrated at seeing so many people wasting their time, energy and hard earned cash on ineffective methods especially diets and plans that only ever have short term success with plenty of negative side effects.

The MSS programme is a real solution. It will be the last book you'll ever need to buy on this topic. However you will need to commit to the programme and follow it exactly step by step. You will not only experience an eye popping body transformation but your life will never be the same again. I can say this with certainty from both personal experience and in witnessing the impact on the lives of thousands of clients worldwide. The fact is that regaining control over your mind/body/health is the catalyst for success in all areas of life. This is why I am so passionate about motivating people just like you to get on the MSS programme as it is a decision that will never stop paying back.

I sit here today writing my story healthy and in a body I feel content with. I feel confident. I have high self esteem with a positive self image. I now love ME and who I am which is the most important thing of all for anyone. However this was not always the case as for the majority of my childhood, teenage years and early adult years I hated myself and my appearance. There were countless nights during this period that I cried myself to sleep. Suicidal thoughts infested my mind much of the time. I hope you don't mind but over the next few pages I am going to share in detail my personal story with you. I do this because I hope you will relate to some of it. I hope that my story will positively impact and inspire you and give you hope and belief that there is always a solution. Also I want to share my journey and story to illustrate that just because I am in great shape, have optimal health and have confidence now that it was not always the case as so many believe. For a long period of my life it could not have been more different.

My Story

Let's go back a few decades so I can share how my life used to be. Between the ages of 9 – 12 I was about 1 and ½ stone (21 Pounds) overweight despite always being active playing sports and just being an active fun loving kid. It was just as well that I was so active. I was eating a reasonably healthy nutrition plan as far as my parents were concerned as it was similar to what most people ate at the time. I dislike using the word diet as you will realise. From about the age of 10 onwards I became self loathing, hating myself and possessing low self esteem. I hated what reflected back at me when I looked in the mirror and I hated what I saw in photos. I became very self conscious. I lacked confidence and possessed an unhealthy disgust in myself, feeling embarrassed by my physical appearance. I felt ugly and totally out of shape despite not even being close to obese. I'll never forget the day my aunt made an issue out of my weight and made me feel terrible telling me to go on a diet. This followed 2 hours mowing her lawn with a push mower in the baking summer heat. To add insult to injury she only gave me a pound which even back then was not a lot for what work I had done!! Just a day later at the age of ten I went on my first "diet" giving up monster munch(crisps) and I haven't eaten them or any crisps since!

Having been a little overweight and self conscious up until around 12 years of age puberty kicked in and there was a total 360 on my appearance. I had a massive growth spurt and seemingly increased metabolism and grew both up and in without changing anything I was doing. I became taller than most of my classmates and friends. I was made feel like I was different and stood out as everyone remarked how tall I was. Now my personal view of myself was a scrawny, skeleton like beanpole. If you know who Mr Bean is (UK comedian and comedy show) then that is what I felt like. Having spent years hating myself for being overweight I now hated myself for the completely opposite reason. I carried these feelings throughout my teenage years – years which were hell for me. When hormones kicked in things went from bad to worse. I felt like the elephant man – not good when you are attracted to most females you see as teenage boys are.

Decades later part of me still cringes when I come across photos from teenage years. One particular photo of a family trip to Amsterdam as we boarded a boat makes me cringe. Even now old emotions are sometimes still stimulated despite now being in such a good place mentally for a number of years. I am now able to look back on this period in my life able to see that there was nothing particularly wrong with me. However in a situation when your perception of yourself is so negative things need to change.

Despite being so skinny I was not lean. I had a persistent layer of fat where my abs were supposed to be!! Nowadays I refer to such body shapes as "Skinny Fat". It is possible to have a high body fat percentage while appearing skinny in clothes.

Teenage years can be tough for many reasons as I am sure you too experienced. I expect that you can appreciate how possessing such a poor self image and having zero confidence made these years 10 times more difficult and mentally tortuous. This was a very difficult phase in my life but now looking back I can see it was a crucial part of my journey through life. If I hadn't experienced it then you wouldn't be reading this book and your life wouldn't be about to change dramatically over the coming weeks.

As well as lacking self confidence I also felt totally unattractive and even ugly(hate that word!). I believed I was never good enough at anything focusing on all things negative. I also believed I would never be good enough for anyone and wouldn't be attractive to anyone. As a result of my scrawny physique sports were challenging. I lacked any physicality. Naturally low self confidence didn't help either. To make matters worse I was an emotionally closed person so I kept my feelings to myself. On the exterior I always appeared happy and was fun to be around. Even from a young age I naturally gravitated towards making people feel better. But when alone I went through hell, often crying myself to sleep and wishing that life would end. I came scarily close on a few occasions to ending it all. Thankfully I didn't and today I look back on my journey as happening for a reason. For a few decades now I have dedicated my life to educating, motivating and inspiring people, just like you, in regaining control over their mind/body/health and ultimately life as a result.

So why is sharing all of this with you relevant to MSS? I am hoping you will relate to some or all of my experiences and that it will inspire you and give you hope. When mentally and emotionally in a dark place you need a ray of light and inspiration and spark to take that first step to change things. My friend, who I will mention soon, and Bill Phillips Body For Life Book were my sparks and ray of hope. You need to find someone who you can relate to. Someone who has succeeded in getting out of a mental black hole. At this moment as you read this book your perception of yourself has hugely impacted your mindset and as a result everything you have done or not done for years. If you feel negative about yourself then you won't attract many positive things into your life and instead negative things, people and experiences. Am I right? This is why I stress in my coaching that regaining control of your mind/body/health is the single most important action one can take. I want to stress to you the importance of achieving YOUR ideal body shape whatever this means to you. Your physical transformation will be the catalyst for success in all areas of life and I have personally experienced this in my own life as well as witnessing it in the lives of thousands of clients all over the world.

The journey I have been on since the age of 9 has lead me to where I am today and formed me into the man I am. I am truly grateful that my life's purpose has been to positively impact the lives of thousands of individuals just like you from all over the world for over 2 decades now. And we are only getting warmed up!! I am grateful to have been able to educate, motivate and inspire others to achieve their own body transformation and as a result experience the positive impact on all areas of their own lives. When my fitness career started at just 17 I promised myself this would be the outcome and reminded myself after becoming Body For Life Champion in 2004. I 100% believe everything happens for a reason and my journey happened for a reason. I am here to change your life forever.

I entered university at just 17 years of age and alcohol became my crutch. It was a form of escapism, a source of false confidence with girls and socially as I partied 4 or 5 nights a week. One day during year 1 a great friend of mine, also Dave, invited me to go to the university gym with him. I had never set foot in a gym and had a very negative perception of what it was like. Spending time in a room with a bunch of knucklehead egotistical bodybuilders was not something I saw as fun. Add to that my certainty of feeling totally inadequate, puny and weak so I turned the offer down. Dave however was a persistent bugger and one day after constant nagging I gave in – being honest just to shut him up – and went to the gym with him. As they say the rest is history. The gym and exercise became my saviour and this is why I am so passionate about sharing my experience and knowledge with as many people like you all over the world as is possible. This is my life's mission and my life's purpose. I am determined for you and others to experience the life changing impact of regaining control over your mind/body/health.

Getting hooked on, and some would say obsessive about, the gym became an important and positive step in my life. I started to feel better about myself and even thought I looked a bit better when looking in the mirror.

This was a good start but like you I then struggled for many years trying everything with minimal results for my effort prior to acquiring the knowledge I will share with you in the Metabolic Stimulation System. Now I am regarded by many as a leading expert in metabolism and body transformation!!

As you read through this book I will give you a full understanding of what your metabolism actually is, how it works, why it is crucial to fat loss/gain and how you too can stimulate it to maximise your fat burning ability. As you read this book it will become crystal clear why everything you have been doing up to this point has been ineffective and in many cases damaging to your metabolism (don't worry the good news is that a slow metabolism can be reversed by the Metabolic Stimulation System). I will reveal to you exactly what the Metabolic Stimulation System is and how you will experience your own body transformation in as little as just 6 weeks!! This book contains your 6 week step by step plan for creating a metabolic furnace so you can start getting lean and sculpted in just weeks. I will be sharing all my secret Metabolic Stimulation System strategies and I expect you to be blown away by the transformation you will experience just as many of our clients around the world have experienced in following the Metabolic Stimulation System programme. I have dedicated every day of my life for over 2 decades to sourcing and acquiring this knowledge and expertise. My mission has always been to serve YOU to the best of my ability providing you with the solutions you need. I am going to share with you how I gained this knowledge and expertise and what I personally had to go through to acquire it. I have been relentless in the pursuit of the most scientific strategies to successfully achieve YOUR ideal body transformation, revealing your abs and importantly easily maintaining control over your mind/body/health forever!!

In just 6 weeks you can completely transform YOUR body, BUT only by following MSS exactly. It works and works faster than anything else out there. Are you still thinking that this is too good to be true? You can see some of our client transformations on the resources page. Here I am, claiming that such results can be achieved in ONLY 6 weeks, when as pointed out earlier you have likely spent years fighting what feels like a lost cause. From my story I hope you now have hope. I hope you now feel that I am the right person to change your results. Remember I personally won my battle and now you too will be armed with the MSS programme which will become a friend for life. I will continue to share my story with you and in doing so illustrate how

(1) I can empathise with your predicament and

(2) I have the knowledge to change your life forever.

I want to stress again that transforming your body is so much more than just looking good. Your mindset will completely change and remember your brain and mindset are your control tower. Regain control and anything is possible. Regaining control of your mind/body/health is the catalyst for success in ALL areas of your life. Keep reminding yourself of this. I sure will be. As I have shared I personally experienced this positive impact as have thousands of my clients around the world. Now it is your turn to experience it. Now is YOUR time. Are you ready?

Today armed to the teeth with knowledge I can look back and clearly see the key role nutrition played throughout my life. Growing up our daily nutrition wasn't terrible as we did eat plenty of fresh healthy food. However much of it was meat and dairy based which over the last 11 years I have grown to learn is a major reason for obesity and the majority of health issues in the world today. Like most who will be reading this book you may be surprised by my claim in the last sentence. However I was the same just over a decade ago now. I am not going to get into this topic now as I go into detail in Section 3 Chapter 8 "Why Plant Based Makes Sense". In that chapter I will share the truth about the negative impact meat and dairy foods have, not just on your fat levels but your health and longevity and not forgetting quality of life.

We regularly ate high-fat and processed foods, sweets, cakes, ice creams etc as was common in most households and still is. Dinner was always followed by a dessert and tea was always accompanied by biscuits. Wouldn't be right otherwise right?? Such was the norm. Such associations are so stupid when you think about them but we are conditioned by brilliant marketing. And there is no one who doesn't like junk food. For many years growing up I also used to drink a litre of coke everyday – not good!! Nowadays along with McDonalds and Pringles it is something I tell people to NEVER have or to let their children have.

I loved toasted cheese sandwiches or cereal late at night watching TV. Do any of these habits/routines sound familiar? It was just as well that I was so active from a young age as otherwise I would have had a real obesity problem. The main problem with my diet during that phase of my life was that it was nutritionally unbalanced, highly toxic and very acidic. I used to eat large quantities too, most of the time as much as any adult.

As previously mentioned I was 17 when the gym became an integral part of my life. It saved me in so many ways. I will always be thankful to Dave for his persistence. Looking back I now know my reluctance to enter the gym was just a get out clause, an excuse and a script I was running in my head. We all have such destructive scripts running in our heads which hold us back from progress and success in any area of life. The real problem was me. I had visualised being this scrawny guy being laughed at doing bicep curls with pathetic 1 Kg dumbbells. I felt intimidated. I felt fear. Can you relate? Or if you have yet to enter a gym for similar reason I bet you can feel the same feelings as I have shared right?

When I commit to something I give it my heart and soul. And the gym and exercise was no different. I trained 3 hours per day including aerobic classes, circuit training, weight lifting, running, and thousands of sit-ups daily. I felt great. I felt fit. I felt myself getting stronger. But much to my frustration and dismay I was only seeing minimal visible difference in my body shape and fat levels particularly around the belly. I could see a level of tone and muscle growth but I wanted more. I wanted abs!! I was baffled as to how, despite all of the time, effort and energy I was putting in, I still had fat covering my sixpack. Surely 3 hours of training a day and thousands of abdominal crunches was enough to get abs? In Section 2 Chapter 3 "Why Ab Crunches Are A Waste Of Time" you will learn why my abs were not becoming visible and why all these crunches made me look fatter not slimmer!!

The ROI (Return On Investment) from my training and nutrition regime was frustrating the hell out of me. I, like anyone reading this book wanted a better body. I wanted a lean sculpted one like you see on the cover of Men's Health. Feeling much fitter and stronger was only a small consolation. When I got hooked on exercise I enrolled to qualify as a fitness trainer. I have always believed that if you put yourself out there as an expert or teacher of anything you should be a role model too. Otherwise in my eyes you have no credibility. You should walk the walk. I was determined to become known worldwide as a top body transformation coach. In my mind people needed to look at me and instantly feel respect and trust that I could deliver the results they wanted.

Once I got into this new "healthy" lifestyle I often cooked my own meals. I rarely had junk food as I got into the weekly "cheat day" mentality and routine. I only drank alcohol at weekends. So what was I doing wrong? What stones was I leaving unturned? This desire to find the solution is what ignited my quest to learn and I was determined to keep searching until I found the solution. Since 1995 I have invested over 100K travelling internationally researching, completing courses, hiring mentors and coaches and learning from the best of the best. I believe in the kaizen method – constant and never ending learning – and continue to practice it today and will until my final days. My huge time and financial investment paid off. I found the solution. That solution is the Metabolic Stimulation System.

As I learned new strategies I became my personal guinea pig. This was my own personal research. If I found something worked I would then incorporate it into client training programmes to see the impact on different body types. I learned that there are 2 crucial factors in achieving fast lasting results :

1. muscle stimulation is a necessity
2. nutrition is 80% of getting results

You will read dedicated chapters in this book on these findings so you can gain a full understanding of why they are so important. The books that I initially learned a lot from were "Body For Life" by Bill Phillips and "High Intensity Training" by Mike Mentzer. What I had been finding in my research was being backed up by the principles being taught in these books. And most importantly they made sense versus all that I had learned in qualifying as an fitness instructor and Personal Trainer. I learned more effective "real life" body transformation strategies in these books than in many of the expensive courses I had invested in. Plain and simple without applying the right level of intensity and without following a balanced nutrition programme you are going nowhere fast. As I implemented my learnings and developed an understanding of the complexity of the human body I realised what an exact science getting lean and muscular actually is. It is far more complex than what is usually recommended which is to just eat less and exercise more. This is fine if obese or just starting out but in order to get really lean and sculpted it takes a precise scientifically based and personalised training and nutrition plan to see results. When I first got into exercise I had been investing a large quantity of time into training but without using effective training principles. I was just doing what others were doing, most of whom looked the same year round. It is amazing to think that in so many situations we do the same thing over and over with same results yet still are reluctant to change. Finally I understood that it is quality not quantity that matters. It takes precision in both your exercise and nutrition to transform your body.

In 2004 I was announced Irish "Body For Life Challenge" Champion. I had reached a bodyfat percentage of just 5% after gaining 26 pounds of muscle and shedding 14 pounds of fat in just 12 weeks. This was a huge milestone and turning point for me. In my own eyes I had graduated to becoming a true role model. The teacher must always lead the way and inspire. I had proven I knew how to achieve what people wanted and since then I have dedicated my life to finding even faster ways as well as sharing this knowledge with my followers and clients worldwide. It is now the latter half of 2016 and I have continued my attitude towards learning and will do so forever. My knowledge continues to expand daily and my clients get the fastest results possible using the most effective strategies which only the minority of coaches are aware of. There is always new research and strategies so the key to being the best is staying ahead and keeping open minded. The training and nutrition programmes my clients now follow are very different to when I first started out as a trainer in 1995, different to 10 years ago and even 5 years ago. My clients and now YOU follow the most effective strategies I know. Follow what I teach and there can only be a positive outcome.

After becoming BFL Champion in 2004, I then coached the "Body For Life" winners for the following five consecutive years. At the time of writing this book I have now coached thousands of people both face to face and online in many countries around the world in achieving the body of their dreams through my strategies. Check out some success stories at the resources page. I have dedicated my life to helping people like you transform their bodies not just fast but so that results are lifelong and are easily maintained. These last 2 words are the most important.

I hope having shared my personal story with you that you now believe that I can truly empathise with your frustrations and how you probably feel like throwing in the towel. You feel like giving up the battle to shed that last layer of fat covering your abs. Don't despair. You are holding the solution right now in your hands (or on your laptop or kindle!). However I must stress that this journey won't be easy. You must be disciplined and follow the programme exactly. To achieve significant results in just 6 weeks there is no room for error. Focus on the prize. How much is it worth to you? How big is your Why?

Don't let this book become a dust collector. Knowledge is not power, implementation of knowledge is power. Taking action is what counts.

My mission is to help you achieve your own transformation – mind/body/health and life. Don't waste any more time, energy or money on diets, gimmicks, fads or average trainers or training systems that promise the world but only deliver disappointment and frustration.

What you have in your hands is invaluable and is the result of 20+ years of my life dedicated to sourcing the most effective strategies to getting in shape, uncovering abs and creating your ideal body shape. This will be the last book of it´s kind you will ever need to buy. I look forward to educating and coaching you over the course of this book. I look forward to reading your success story which I would love you to share with us via one of our social media channels or in our private MSS facebook group.

Now let's start the education process and then after that get into the nitty gritty of exactly what you need to do step by step for the next 6 weeks.

Section 1 : Mindset

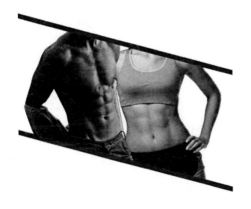

1 – If You Don't Know Where You're Going How Can You Get There?

Understand this – Unless you train your mind, as regularly as you train your body, success will never, I repeat NEVER be achieved. What you believe in your mind and how truly you believe it will determine whether you will achieve it or not.

The fact that you are reading this book right now is proof that you want to improve your body, yourself and your life. However have you ever taken the time to clarify 100% in your mind and on paper what you want to ultimately achieve? What is success to you? Can you describe to me right now in detail what I would see in front of me when you have finally achieved your goal?

TAKE NOTE : I advise you to write goals in ink versus typing on a laptop using a word doc. It has been scientifically proven that the process of physically writing something down imprints it more on your mind and subconscious.

If you have never invested the time and energy into clarifying your desired outcome then this is one of the main reason why you have spent years or possibly decades on this seemingly never ending, unrewarding and unsuccessful journey to achieve your ideal body shape. Napoleon Hill made a great statement in Think

And Grow Rich (while it is a book more about professional and financial success the same principles apply to all areas of life). He stated that you must "See, Feel and Believe Yourself Already In Possession Of Your Goal". This is a powerful statement. If you can't visualise your outcome and if you don't fuly believe in your ability to achieve your goal success will be impossible. Why? Because subconsciously you are already beaten and your subconscious will ultimately direct your thoughts and actions. It is why so many people spend their entire lives experiencing the same cycle of success and then failure with every weight loss group or system they join. They are beaten subconsciously before they even attended the first meeting. Feeling a glimmer of hope was all that got them to start.

You must be clear on your desired outcome. You must have laser focus on your desired outcome. However most importantly you must believe that you are going to achieve it and make it reality. Now none of this is easy but this is why the first section of this book is all about mindset. You must create a positive mental environment creating positive energy and excitement around your goal. You must create a mindset that believes it is a matter of WHEN you are going to achieve your goal not IF!! When I made my decision to enter The Body For Life Challenge I also made the decision that I needed to win it and become champion. I decided on what my outcome needed to be statistically and aesthetically to become champion and then drew up my plan of action to take me from point A to B. Once I had done this I knew 100% that once I followed through on my plan, taking each step and gave it 100% I would become champion. I saw myself as champion months before being announced as I visualised my desired outcome a few times a day. I took time daily to engage my senses and feel what the moment would be like when I was announced as champion. I believed 100% that all I needed to do was follow the plan I had laid out and I would achieve my goal. In achieving any goal you must be 100% clear and definite about your point B. Once you know your point A and B you can then decide what steps are required along the journey to have a successful trip. Make sense?

If like most people you have never fully clarified your goals then what follows is your crucial first step before you even think about exercise and nutrition. Your chances of achieving your ideal body shape and optimal health depend on what you do next. Without clarity on your goal how do you expect to get there? You don`t even know where you want to go. Even having the best tools available to you, like Metabolic Stimulation System, will be useless if you aren't clear on where you want to end up – make sense? So as our first step on your MSS journey let's focus on your point B – where exactly do you want to end up?

Now you may be surprised that we are not focusing on your point A. You may be surprised that we are not focusing on all the reasons why you hate yourself right now and why your body and life has to change. This may seem strange and counter-intuitive from what you have read in many other body transformation books or heard from other "experts" but in my personal opinion they take the totally wrong approach. It is commonly thought in popular media, books and among many "experts" that in order to move away from our pain we must focus on it. We must focus on all the pain it is causing us and that will stimulate us to take drastic action to change our situation. I totally disagree with this approach and feel it is why millions have only ever gone so far in their body transformation efforts. It completely creates the wrong energy around the goal. There is so much more benefit and power in creating positive energy around a goal and project. It is much more beneficial to create excitement about the future you vs dwelling on the pain of why you feel miserable and hate yourself at this precise moment and likely have done for a long time. Positive energy creates. Negative energy destroys. In a body transformation scenario negative energy ensures short term success and eventual failure.

Let's test my train of thought. Sit down on a comfortable seat or on the floor or lie down. Get a comfortable positive and close your eyes. Take a minute now to visualise yourself in your ideal body shape. Scan your whole body as if looking through the eyes of another person. Become aware of your senses and really feel the emotions running through your body both in how you feel and in the admiring glances of others. Feel the positive energy from the smile on your face and the confidence that is oozing. Sense how you feel about yourself at this moment in your ideal body shape. How good does it feel to have a positive self image, good self esteem and to feel good about yourself and your body?

Did that simple exercise make you feel good even though it hasn't happened yet? But you got a sense of hope that it will become reality right? This is the power of putting a focus on creating positive energy. Our thoughts and actions are all driven by our emotions and feelings. Therefore it is crucial that we start by making you feel positive, excited and even feel a little belief that your goal will be a reality by following my Metabolic Stimulation System. Are you starting to feel this?

Now let's make a decision on your outcome – your point B. There are 3 important elements :

1. **Have a clearly defined goal :** detailed description of your outcome. Be able to clearly describe to someone what they will see when they see you. What are the key features? What stands out? What are the differences compared to now? What reflects from the mirror as you stand there naked in front of it?

2. **Have a measurable goal :** be able to prove your success via indicators like body fat percentage using a skinfold calipers, tape measurements, clothes size, photos, energy levels, strength/fitness challenges etc You need indicators that you can measure right now, during and at the end so you can track your progress along the way and prove your goal been achieved statistically at the end as well as what you can see and feel. So decide on what your end statistics are going to be, based on what vision you have for #1 above.

3. **Have a realistic goal :** NOTE – this is not in terms of the realistic expectations of others as they will either see your desired outcome being way below your capabilities or they will just put your goals down from the start. What I mean here is that the target you set is realistic in that you can achieve it in the timespan you are allowing for it. For example when I started my Body For Life Challenge I set myself what others would have considered a totally unrealistic

target. With my body type packing on the level of muscle I required to have a chance of winning was a major challenge. It meant beating my genetics. For many it appeared an impossible challenge but I proved them wrong and gained 26 pounds of lean muscle in just 12 weeks finishing at 5% bodyfat. It pushed me to my very limits but I did it. Now if I had aimed to pack on 50 pounds of muscle in 12 weeks that would have been unrealistic – make sense? So push your limits and your imagination and make yourself feel uncomfortable about the goal you set but make sure it is possible.

Now let's talk about goal statements as I want you to use steps #1 to #3 above to write your own personal goal statement. Setting goal statements like " I want to have a six pack" or "I want to get in great shape" are way too vague. You need to be way more specific. Remember in the last exercise I wanted you to visualise exactly what you will look like and decide on what your final statistics would likely be. What bodyfat % do you need to be in order to look as you will in point B? How are you going to measure success? What will be your exact body fat %, weight, tape measurements, clothes size for both upper and lower body, level of energy, daily emotions, quality of sleep etc. What measurements matter to you? Include mentions of them in your goal statement. What will your new self-image feel like? How are you going to feel? Such measurements create clarity and focus. Also make sure to write your goal statement in the present tense as this keeps imprinting on your brain what will happen every time you read it. Turn a goal like "I am in great shape and feel good" into "I am 12 stone and currently at

13% bodyfat, have a 34 inch waist and I woke up this morning before my alarm feeling fresh and alert". This is clearly defined. This is measurable. This is realistic. Begin with the end in mind. Take time now to think about what you want your outcome to be and then WRITE IT DOWN in the space provided under "goal statement" in the **Tools & Resources Section** at the back of the book.

NOTE : I want you to dream big and let your imagination go wild. But be realistic as mentioned above. To help you in determining your goal here is a guideline. For example if you are male or female, 20 stone or more and at a 35% bodyfat or more you will not reveal your abs in 6 weeks. But in 6 months you sure will.

Revealing abs means achieving a body fat percentage of 10% or lower for a male and 18-20% or lower for a female. So if you are already lean, around the body fat percentage of 15% (male) or 25% (female) then after this 6 week MSS Program you can definitely have achieved <10% male or < 18% female and have visible abs.

Now that you have clearly written down your goal statement you should find it easier to visualise your desired outcome. I want you to make a promise to yourself now that you will commit just 5 minutes daily to visualisation. Decide on whether you will do your daily visualisation session first thing each morning after waking or last thing at night before going to sleep. If you have the discipline to fit it in do it both times as there is no better way to start or finish your day. It is important that you schedule this into your daily routine as unless you plan action it won't happen. Remember as I mentioned earlier you need to "see, feel and believe yourself already in possession of the goal" as Napoleon Hill said. Visualisation is a key strategy in creating this mindset. Commit to this daily practice now.

Now let's focus again on creating some positive energy and excitement about your goal. What is your why? What positive impact will your new mind/body/health have on all areas of your life? Your why must be strong to inspire and motivate you to be willing to do anything to achieve your goal. You must create a burning desire. You must feel excited each time you think of your goal and demonstrate the determination and passion required to succeed. You must create a mindset which will not even contemplate the possibility of failure. Your why list in combination with the exercises we have already gone through in this chapter will ensure this. Answer the following questions :

- What areas of your life will be most positively impacted by your new body shape, positive mindset and optimal health?
- How will feeling confident impact your decision making?
- How will feeling confident, sexy and attractive impact your relationships in general and intimately with your partner? Or even in your comfort in getting out socially and making the first move if single?
- How will control over your body/mind/health impact your professional life and in achieving your professional ambitions?
- What impact will having boundless energy and vitality have on your life?

- How will you feel hitting the beach or the pool in your new lean sculpted body?

Take time to write out your Why List. Think about all the wonderful benefits and experiences your new body and life will bring with them. Just focus on writing and don't think too much. Let them flow out of you. Let your heart drive your writing hand until you run out of whys. Go to the Tools & Resources to fill in your Why List – there are 50 spaces – and to see the link to download a Why List sheet to fill in should you prefer.

How did you feel going through the process of writing your Why List? Make you smile? Feel excited? Energetic? Positive? Clients typically do when we do this exercise. You are getting a sense of the feelings and emotions you will possess when you achieve your goal. Now what is really important is that you regularly remind yourself of your why list. You must regularly remind yourself of all that awaits you from following the Metabolic Stimulation System. I am excited about how much your life will have changed just 6 weeks from now. You should be excited too. It is the start of a journey that will change your life forever.

Next let's talk about taking photos. Photos are a powerful tool both for motivation and tracking progress. Before starting the 6 week programme take your photos – front, back and side view – in bikini/swimsuit(ladies) and shorts(guys) and stick copies of them where you will regularly see them. Then take photos at the end of each week in the same swimming costume and compare them. Why are photos powerful tools? Photos don't lie. When you look at yourself in the mirror your perception of what you are seeing is formed by your state of mind at the time. If in a good mood you will see progress a lot easier than if having a bad day when you will likely see yourself at your worst. You cannot alter what looks back from a photo in any way. Make sense? Also by taking photos each week it allows you to become aware of the speed of progress. You will be able to see whether any tweaks may be needed in your training or nutrition programme to accelerate results. This is why logging everything is also important as I will stress in Section 2 and 3 on exercise and nutrition. There is no time to lose.

Another angle with the use of photos I want you to use is to have a photo representing your 6 week goal. This can either be a previous picture of yourself when you were in your ideal shape or can be a photo of someone's body you want to replicate. Remember we want to create positive energy and belief about the outcome you are going to achieve. Keep this photo in your diary, on your fridge, screensaver on computer even in your wallet. Don't miss any chance to reinforce and hit your subconscious with a physical visual of what you want to look like. Create this mental image. Reinforce your belief that in 6 weeks you will have a dramatic change to your body and lifestyle.

Next you need to measure your weight, bodyfat percentage (with a skinfold callipers) and tape measurements taken. If any of these are not possible that is fine. Clothes and photos will show progress as well as you knowing yourself. However the tape measurements should be possible for anyone. I am not a big fan of weighing scales and only include it here as I know many will track it even if I say not to. It is up to you but just remember that your weight is impacted by many factors so is not a reliable indicator of progress. For the tape measurements I want you to take in the following places :

Chest/back – starting at mid chest (between breasts for a lady) and go all the way around

Waist – start at belly button and go all the way round

Hips (just women) – widest part and all the way round

Arms : mid upper arm and around

Thighs : Mid upper thigh and around

Fill in your starting measurements in the Progress Tracker in the Tools & Resources section at the back of the book. You can also download a Progress Tracker there too. Take your measurements weekly, fill in your progress tracker and review them gauging whether results are on track to achieve your desired outcome. It is critical to use such tools to measure progress. Use the information from these measurements and your training and nutrition logs to plan the following week. Go to the Tools and Resources section for your training and nutrition logbooks.

At this stage you have 2 powerful motivational tools

1. written material i.e. your goal and why list and
2. Goal photo

And various progress indicator as we have just outlined.

Next let's identify aspects of your current lifestyle that need to be accounted for in designing your personalised programme. Creating a healthy active lifestyle is about setting realistic goals based on what consumes each 24 hours of your day. We all get the same amount of time each day but we all have different commitments and priorities each day. And we are all different at how productive we are and how effectively we use the time we have. Planning and preparation are key to success. What aspects of your lifestyle currently consume time that are fixed, breakable or unexpected? Also these can be elements of your current lifestyle that impact what you can do with regard to exercise and possibly nutrition.

Fixed obstacles include working hours, set time commitments, injury, disability etc. None are excuses but you must work around these. Breakable obstacles such as your social life, tv, time online using social media, recreational activities, current level of motivation, knowledge, cooking experience, reaction of family and friends can be altered in your time commitment to them and in how much you prioritise them. This is the area that people are wasting a lot of time and energy and could be doing more to better position themselves for success. With regard to unexpected obstacles just identify potential obstacles and plan for them. Look back on the last few months and identify unexpected obstacles that potentially could reoccur. Be prepared for what life has to throw at you as life will always throw challenges but embrace them as each one is a learning opportunity.

Chapter Summary and Action Steps :

- Become 100% laser focused and clear on your goal and write down your goal statement

- Commit to 5 minutes daily visualisation. Either first thing each morning on waking or last thing at night before sleeping or both times.
- Create emotional intensity and positive energy towards your goal by writing your why list focusing on all the wonderful experiences and benefits of following the programme
- Take your "before" photos and take new photos at the end of each week. Also select or create a point B photo that illustrates your goal. Remind yourself of these photos throughout each day and place in prominent positions so you will see them regularly. Attach your photos to the allocated pages in the Tools and Resources section at the back of the book.
- Take your starting tape measurements and ideally your body fat percentage if possible using a skinfold calipers. Decide your measurement goals for the end of week 6. Fill in your progress tracker at the end of each week.
- Identify what aspects of your current lifestyle need to be planned for as well as what current habits can you change to buy back time and create more positive energy.

2 – Belief Is The Thin Line Between Success And Failure

I want to ask you 2 questions and I want you to be 100% honest in your answers :

1. When planning goals do you typically aim safe and keep within what you feel is realistic?

2. Do you often change your goals, aiming lower as a result of being influenced by the reactions of others after you have shared your goals with them?

If you answered Yes to one or both questions then we need to revise your goal statement from chapter 1 as well as working harder on your mindset. This will hopefully prevent you from falling into the trap of question 2!! I want you to dream as big as you can. You can achieve the body shape you want to see reflecting back from the mirror. You can be anything you want in life. You can achieve anything that you want in life. Showing a burning desire and determination in combination with taking consistent positive progressive action is what achieves success. It is YOUR life and YOUR dream so live fully without being limited by boundaries you are creating in your mind.

It is now time to make your dreams reality. However in order to succeed in regaining control of your mind/body/health it is crucial that you create a mental environment where you believe 100% that success is the only possible outcome. Once you truly believe you will achieve.

There is actual a very thin line between those who succeed and those who don't. Everyone has dreams and goals and most take action to some degree. Most make an attempt to better their lives. But only the minority take consistent action for the necessary time it takes to succeed. These people deal with life's curveballs and challenges and meet them head on and dust themselves off and move on. Such people have impenetrable belief that they will succeed. It is just a matter of when not if and they are determined to find the quickest route there. On the flip side the majority of people don't possess this belief and stop taking action before they get to their outcome. They hope their dreams are going to just happen if they wish for them hard enough. It is the lottery mentality. These people aren't willing to put in the work. They tell themselves they are stuck in the body they have. They blame their genetics. They blame their thyroid. They blame their lifestyle. They never stay focused and take consistent action. They never take responsibility. Why? What is the main difference here between such people and those who do succeed? Belief.

Once you decide on a clear picture of your goal and start taking consistent action your hope turns into belief. You start to see results. Your level of belief is the thin line between success and failure – that is all!! If you keep generating positive energy through consistent action, results and daily mindset training you will start to truly believe in yourself, your goal and your ability to transform your body and life. Sadly many who "fail" are within touching distance of succeeding when they stop taking action. For whatever reason they lost hope and desire at the crucial moment despite progress being before them but they could not see it. Maybe it was lack of understanding through poor education of how things work creating unrealistic expectations. Maybe it was down to constant negativity from family and "friends" and colleagues that finally wore them down. You must never give up. You must believe in your goal. Successful people in all walks of life prove the power of consistent action and belief. You are no different to them – flesh and bones but is your mind consumed with desire and belief? Or doubt and negativity? This is the thin line you must cross. Your mind is the control tower – remember that.

Another important difference with people who successfully transform their bodies and lives is that challenges and "failures" are embraced and met head on not frowned upon. You need to change your mindset around challenges. "Failures" are learning experiences. You can learn from every experience regardless of whether at the time it is perceived good or bad. Once you implement new learnings you will move on a stronger more powerful individual. Such a mentality is crucial in any journey, body transformation or otherwise. No goal is easily come by and life is always full of ups and downs. Don't expect your journey over the next 6 weeks to be plain sailing. Don't wait for a 6 week period that you think you have a "clear run". There is no "best time" to follow a programme. The time is always now as there will be no straightforward challenge free journey to your body transformation over the next 6 weeks or beyond.

You must prove how much you want success and keep working on creating a positive mindset – one that is a positive focused mental environment.

In most sports, at the highest level, there is very little difference in ability between the winners and the losers. It is those who believe in themselves and their vision the most who will be victorious. The winners are often the ones who have visualised themselves winning more than anyone else. And importantly they have believed in the vision they have seen in their mind. This is why you will hear me refer to visualisation many times during this section of the book as it is a key part of a mindset training programme. The power of mental training is totally underestimated and is even more powerful than your physical training. Without the right mindset you will never adhere to your training and nutrition programme. When life throws challenges or someone gives you a nasty comment there will be a strong possibility that you will give up or take the foot off the pedal. As a result you will never taste success. Don't let this happen. Create a success mindset and follow the Metabolic Stimulation System programme exactly step by step as outlined.

Inevitably there are going to be days where training is the last thing you want to do. There will be days you feel like breaking your nutrition programme too. There will be days where you just want to give up on that last repetition when your muscles are burning, or stop when your lungs feel like exploding during cardio HIIT training. You are a human being run by your emotional state. No one likes discomfort no matter what the benefits may be. And it is all the more difficult to adhere to a programme when negative emotions are winning the battle in your mind. However this is where your burning desire is being tested. How much do you really want this? Win this battle consistently.

Regardless of what you think of his doping scandal this is a great quote, which I love, by Lance Armstrong

"Winners never quit and quitters never win"

Your split second decisions will play a key role in your success or failure. You must learn to react positively to the negative voices in your head. There is a lazy bad guy in your head that doesn't have your best interests at heart. Ignore him. Believe in yourself. Believe in your potential. It is truly unlimited!!

To achieve the results that are possible following the Metabolic Stimulation System you must push your limits and regularly smash your comfort zone. Realise that physically you have no limits. You are only limited by self imposed limits you may have in your head or by listening to the opinion of others. The human body has the amazingly ability to adapt to any stress and stimulation applied whether it is a good or bad stress. Promise yourself that you won't become one of the majority who hold back or worse still give up when the going gets tough. You are made of sterner stuff than that. Believe it. Don't give up just at the point when you will stimulate your body to new growth. Push through your pain thresholds. Focus on the many carrots that await you by achieving this goal.

Have you a support network or are you your sole supporter? Have you previously experienced progress only to revert back to old habits again as a result of the reaction of others? Do you allow yourself to be influenced to eat unhealthy food or to skip exercise? Have you experienced being told that you were boring as a result of following a healthier and more active lifestyle? One of the most crucial action steps you can take in life in general is to take a good look at the people around you. Are they the type of people who will support and encourage you? Who will celebrate your successes? Who will champion you and push you to keep going when you feel like quitting? The people in your life right now are going to have a crucial impact on your level of success with Metabolic Stimulation System so you need to make sure they are the right type. If you are keeping company with unhealthy, inactive, lazy, obese negative individuals then it will be incredibly difficult for you to get in the best shape of your life. When you start moving outside someone's comfort zone they will try to pull you back in. This is very evident when it comes to body and health as everyone wants change in this area but only a minority are willing to put in the work required. It is very important to take some time to look at your family and current friends and decide if they are suitable to what you need in your circle. This can be a tough and emotional exercise for many. However if change is required it will be the most important decision you will make. It will be the difference between your success and failure. Prioritise surrounding yourself with people congruent with your goals and possessing the right characteristics and lifestyles to support and motivate you.

A lack of belief is heavily evident in anyone possessing a negative mindset. Possessing a positive mindset is crucial and it is key that you fill your mind and life with positive energy. Commit on a daily basis to read, watch, and listen to self growth, personal development and positive energy material. Decide what motivates and inspires you. Surround yourself with the right people. Limit your exposure to those who are toxic in your life and even eliminate people where needed. Identify those individuals that most inspire and uplift you and spend more time with them and start bringing them into your inner circle. I encourage you to include a daily mental training programme as I share in this section such as reading your goals, reading your why list, visualisation and personal development work. It is about creating new positive habits that become part of your lifestyle where you don't have to consciously decide to do it similar to brushing your teeth or sleeping. Mental training is a key piece of the formula in regaining control of your mind/body/health.

In summary increasing your belief and consistent positive reinforcement are crucial daily activities. You must believe that success will be the only outcome. There is a thin line between success and failure which is ultimately determined by your mindset and the level of belief you have in achieving your goal. If you truly believe in your goal, then it will happen. Make sure you take that step across the thin line. Also take time to review your current circle of people in your life. Identify those who you need to either eliminate completely or limi your exposure to. You need to have positive influences in your life who will encourage you towards your goals.

3 – See, Feel and Believe Yourself Already In Possession Of Your Goal

In the previous two chapters you set your goals and identified potential obstacles. You were also introduced to the importance of daily mental training and how you must really believe that you will achieve your goal. This chapter will work on developing your belief further. Developing a positive mindset is a critical part of the Metabolic Stimulation System as I have stressed a number of times so far. I personally include time for mindset training each and every day. It is a key daily habit in my life and needs to be one of yours too. While most clients are usually surprised that I spend so much time on mindset when they start working with me they all point to it as the key factor in their success.

Answer these questions:

- can you see yourself with a toned midsection with visible abs?
- If you are a mother can you see yourself getting your pre childbirth stomach back?
- Can you see yourself feeling comfortable and confident walking along the beach with your ideal body shape, feeling 100% content with your physique, feeling sexy and attractive?

As I mentioned in a previous chapter Napoleon Hill stated that you must

"See, feel, and believe yourself already in possession of your goal."

For you to succeed with Metabolic Stimulation System you must first truly believe in the outcome and keep it's image foremost in your mind. You must truly believe that you are going to achieve your ideal body shape and as time goes on be able to more and more vividly visualise yourself already in possession of your goal.

You committed in a previous chapter to 5 minutes of daily visualisation. If right now you find it difficult to visualise yourself in your ideal body and if when you visualise the picture is unclear or feels forced don't worry. This is normal for everyone at first. Visualisation is a practice no different to yoga, meditation or even exercise. You must develop the skill to do it effectively and to get the most from it. Right now what matters most is that you consistently complete your daily 5 minutes. As you progress through your journey, following the programme, your visualisation experience will become clearer, more visual, and more real similar to when deeply dreaming during sleep. As you experience results over the next 6 weeks your belief will grow stronger. As your belief grows so too will how vividly you visualise.

When visualising choose a quiet location. Close your eyes, put on relaxing music, and bring your point B into your mind and focus on what's happening when Point B is achieved and the feelings you'll experience at that time.

See yourself walking around in the body shape you want. Feel your new energy, vitality and good health. Become aware of the environment surrounding you and become aware of everything around you in this perfect setting. Become aware of your senses. See your ideal life in your ideal body. Conduct this exercise for 5 minutes before slowly opening your eyes. Most successful people are dedicated to their daily visualization. Most successful athletes use visualization. The person whose mind is fixed and focused on their goal, and truly believes in achieving it, is the person who will succeed. Soon this will be you!

Next I want you to write out your success scene. A 'success scene' is a written form of visualisation of your desired outcome with gratitude built into your statement. Write your statement in the present tense detailing the scene – what you have achieved, how you feel, how you look, what you are doing, what you are grateful for, the surroundings etc For example :

"It is the 15th August 10am and I am lying on Flamingo beach where I live in Lanzarote. I can feel the soft sand underneath me. Just 6 weeks ago I started the Metabolic Stimulation System programme. I can hardly believe my eyes as I now look at my tight toned body particularly my midsection where I can see visible abs for the first time in my life. I am so grateful for the support that I received from my family and friends in achieving this goal. I feel amazing. I feel so attractive and sexy in my new body. I finally have a positive self image and high self-esteem. I feel like a new person and that anything I want to achieve is now possible. I am so grateful for what I have achieved."

This is just a brief example of the type of thing you can write out so I hope it gives you an idea of what I want you to do. Can you see how including a concentrated focus on this success scene in your daily mental training will increase your belief that success can be the only outcome. Positive mindfeed is what you want each and every day.

Another tool I advise you to use is a goal card. Write your goal statement as agreed in Chapter 1 onto a card. Start with "I am grateful that..." and finish the statement with your goal written in present tense. Include detail of what you have achieved including a date. Remember in chapter 1 I spoke about goals being clearly defined, measurable and realistic. Keep your goal card in your pocket, so that every time you touch it, you will be reminded of what is written on the card. Your mind will flash images onto your mind.

In summary, it is critical to create a mental environment, where success is the only outcome and you see, feel, and believe yourself already in possession of your goal. Be diligent with your daily mental training regime.

- Read your goal card daily
- Read your why list daily
- Read your success scene daily
- Visualise for a minimum of 5 minutes daily

These habits are an important part of the Metabolic Stimulation System.

Remember I have said that I focus not just on fast results but lifelong results. By creating these habits every day during your 6 week journey you will create positive lifelong habits that will serve you forever whatever your goals may be. So make sure you do these exercises once a day but if you want to push yourself do them twice daily if you feel disciplined enough – first thing in the morning and last thing at night. I start off my day really positively, and I end my day really positively and in my sleep dream about my goals becoming reality. Believe in your mind and make reality through consistent positive progressive action.

4 – Leave No Stone Unturned

It is crucial that you add some urgency to your 6 week journey that is about to start. Treat these 6 weeks like your life depends on it as getting serious for a minute it may do. In the coming years and decades your health and self image will have a big impact on all the decisions you make and your quality of life as it is that serious that you regain control over your mind/body/health. These 6 weeks will be your launchpad to experiencing this. Being such a short period of time there is no room for error or half hearted attempts over the next 6 weeks. Now let's go back to my constant mentions so far in this book of the importance of focusing on creating a long term lifestyle. This certainly is our goal. However we want the next 6 weeks to be a major kickstart for the rest of your life so I want you to really give the next 6 weeks some serious oomph. In order to maximise your results you need to schedule a review and planning session at least once a week. I recommend you do this on sundays after your training/nutrition plan is completed. Benjamin Franklin stated it a long time ago but it still rings true and always will

'If you fail to plan,
you plan to fail'

I recommend that you block off 30 to 60 minutes each sunday to review the week just finished and plan for the week that is about to start. You will be able to identify what is working for you as well as what you are finding challenging and then you can tweak the plan where needed. Lifestyle creation is about finding what works for you personally. Everyone's life is different and we all have different daily and weekly commitments that must be allowed for. A weekly review will provide you with valuable information ensuring optimum progress towards your desired outcome.

I have already stressed how important regaining control of your mind/body/health is a number of times. This is why I want you to create some urgency and create positive energy through excitement and anticipation not stress. I want you to leave no stone unturned in the pursuit of your outcome. A weekly review and planning session must become a habit like the other habits we have discussed so far in this book. The next 6 weeks is long enough to achieve incredible results and embed positive lifelong habits. But also six weeks is short enough to pass you by leaving you with regrets.

The one thing you should fear in life is regret

Please take note of this important sentence – probably the most important one in this book and any book you will read. Make the most of every second, every minute, every hour, every day, every week of the next six weeks and become very conscious of living with this attitude beyond the next 6 weeks. Carry this momentum on for the rest of your life. Once you get into this healthy active new lifestyle the alternative will no longer make any sense.

I would recommend that you log everything. You should have a log for training, nutrition, daily emotions, sleep and a general journal. As well as accelerating results it also allows you to get to know you better and in time to become the real you or return to who you used to be as life and trauma may have seen you lose yourself. Allocate just 10 to 15 minutes each night to fill your logs and use this information to review and plan the following day. Just block this time each evening and make it a part of your daily routine. I would advise you to review and plan your training sessions both during and after training sessions. I do both. During my workout rest periods I record what I have done and compare it to what I had planned. I then plan my next training session while the memory of it's difficulty level and pain are still fresh in my mind. I believe that during workouts is the most effective time to plan your next training session.

Your nutrition log should also show a planned versus actual. Record times, food sources, quantities, feelings after eating and even what company you had if any for each meal. This information will assist you to stay on track. You might notice a trend that you eat certain foods with certain company. Analyse and learn and make changes where beneficial.

Each day record and analyse your emotions. During the day how did you feel? Did you feel aggravated, or have a bad temperament today? Were you very reactive to situations? Did you feel energetic? Tired/lethargic? Happy? Slim/fat? Your mood and emotions will have a big impact on your feelings and your motivation to take action. Remember your thoughts lead to pictures which lead to feelings/emotions which lead to actions which lead to results. This is why it is so crucial for us to have some influence over our thoughts and more importantly how we react to them.

You may not know it but your nutritional choices play a key role in your daily emotions. The food and liquids you consume cause chemical reactions inside you. They impact your blood sugar levels and also how you feel. Some foods effect your hormone levels both in release and suppression. Your brain consumes 20% of the calories you consume daily so remember this when making your food choices. When training consistently and seeing progress as well as predominantly eating wholefoods you will feel amazing, positive and calm. People will enjoy being in your company more. The control you have over your nutrition and training will be reflected in your temperament and mood.

I would also advise you to log your sleeping patterns. You will learn more about the importance of sleep in section 4. Sleep is a crucial part of the whole formula. Your sleep quality determines the speed your muscles recovery from training. There are key steps to take to ensure quality sleep so please implement what is laid out for you step by step in Section 4. Logging your sleep patterns is crucial if you have sleep problems. Like any problem it requires reflection and identifying triggers and becoming aware of the cause. When you know the cause you can then focus on prevention. This applies to everything that requires a solution. Each day ask yourself :

Did I wake up fresh before the alarm or did I hit the snooze button a few times?

Did I fall asleep easily or was I twisting and turning for hours?

Did I sleep through the night, or wake up several times? If so, why ?

Did I feel fresh and energetic all day or lethargic with a major mid afternoon slump?

You should be answering yes to each of these questions. Even if following an effective training and nutrition programme such as Metabolic Stimulation System poor sleeping habits will lead to minimal results.

Take time each night to plan the following day based on the information in your logbooks. Identify potential obstacles and commitments you must keep. Treat each day like a jigsaw and fit in all the pieces. Identify the priorities and these become pieces of that day's jigsaw you must fit in. Exercise, nutrition, quality sleep and mindset should be core foundational pieces in each and every day.

Stay laser focused during this initial 6 week journey and make every second count. Leave no stone unturned, have no regrets and be clear that daily planning and review sessions will be crucial to revealing those abs.

Chapter Key Points & Action Steps :

- If You Fail To Plan You Plan To Fail
- Keep a log of everything each day – your nutrition, exercise, sleep and mood
- Take time to review your logs and make changes where needed
- The only fear you should have in life is REGRET

Section 2 : Exercise

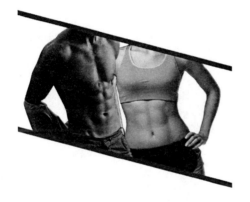

1 – Are You Tough Enough?

As we kick off Section 2 of Metabolic Stimulation System, which will focus on the exercise part of the success formula, I want to ask you what your current body shape is? Are you obese? A bit overweight? In good shape but no visible abs yet? What is your starting point? You may already be in what is considered good shape but not to the level you are aiming for. You may train consistently and eat mainly healthy food while you follow a strict nutrition plan. You may have made many sacrifices for weeks, months or even years in your pursuit of your "Ideal Body". However despite your consistent efforts that lean sculpted body is still just a dream. An aspiration. Right now you feel frustrated at how little return you are gaining from your efforts. Am I right? This is why you are reading my book. Whatever your body shape at this moment it is your starting point. Your experiences up to this point while super frustrating contain lessons. They illustrate to you what definitely does not work and possibly a few things that maybe have but you weren't consistent enough in following them. Each individual will be different but majority who read this book will have followed diets and ineffective exercise programmes. At a time when there has never been so much information available to people like yourself about exercise and nutrition there has never been so much confusion. My aim with MSS is to clarify what actually works, answer questions you have possibly had unanswered for years and to lay out a step by step plan that you can easily follow. My goal is to clarify everything for you by educating you versus just telling you what to do. When you understand the why for anything you are always more likely to do it once it makes sense. I want you to know the why for everything that I am going to ask you to do. Before I educate you about "what effective exercise is" in this section's chapters I need to ask you an important question:

How much do you really want this?

Have you a burning desire to succeed? If so how intense is it? What would being in your ideal body mean to you? Is losing fat, becoming leaner and more sculpted the most important goal in your life right now? If you are not in control of the mind/body/health area of your life then it should be. I can promise you that achieving "your" ideal body shape will be the catalyst for success in all areas of your life. I will continue to stress just how big an impact regaining control of your mind/body/health will have on your life as a whole, throughout this book as I want it to sink in. Your self image and mindset impacts everything that you think, feel and do. I have another question for you:

Are you tough enough for this?

You will need to be.

That may seem like a strange question to ask but you are about to take on your body in the battle of all battles. Let me explain. I am sure you are baffled that over the years all your effort have not paid off. Correct? When one is obese or very overweight you lose "weight" relatively fast when you start a new "diet" and exercise programme. Motivation is high. However as time goes on and you are getting closer to your goal, gaining hope and belief, a similar level of effort and sacrifice yields little or no results. This is where frustration usually kicks in and most give up and revert to previous bad habits. Sound familiar? When you reach a certain point where you are no longer obese or very overweight **your body has no need** to lose more weight/fat or to gain muscle mass. You are no longer carrying a level of fat that may lead to health conditions. Progressing further becomes more about your personal goals vs your body's need to be a certain shape. It is a stage of body transformation which is more about getting leaner for vanity purposes and for aesthetics – make sense?

You are not in your "ideal body shape". You want to look better while many may think you look good. You want to feel better within yourself and more feel more confident. When you reach this plateau or sticking point I referred to earlier your self image and self confidence will be much improved but you need and want more. Here is the challenge and why you need to be tough enough at this point – your body doesn't NEED to lose more fat and it doesn't NEED to pack on more muscle. Of course there are benefits to doing so but your body doesn't NEED it for health purposes. Make sense? You want to look better. You want higher self esteem and a better self image. You want a body that will turn heads, and be the envy of others. There is nothing wrong with this. We all want to look great and turn heads whether we are willing to admit it or not. We live in a very image focused world.

What matters most is that you feel good within yourself and love yourself and having your "ideal body" is key to this.

Besides vanity and self image reasons maybe you need to achieve your ideal body shape because it will have an impact on achieving your professional aspirations and dreams. Maybe you are an athlete who needs to take your athletic performance to the next level to move from amateur to professional. Whatever your why and motivation show the desire to do what it takes to achieve your goal.

Get ready for the ultimate battle between you and your body. Despite going through many periods of sweat and pain in the gym, following diets feeling deprived every day, sacrificing your favourite foods, limiting your social life and prioritising getting in shape and losing weight you are still not in your "ideal body". To achieve your goal you need to be tough enough as reaching your point B will take much more focus and structure with a smarter more effective regime such as Metabolic Stimulation System.

It is a myth that you can just exercise more and eat healthier and get in great shape. It is a lot more complex and scientific and harder than this simple idea. There is no one who is in great shape that did this. Is there anything in life that is worth achieving that is easy? That just takes a small bit of effort? Anyone lean and muscular all gave 100% and met physical and mental challenges daily to get there. It is far from easy but this is where desire comes in. Achieving your ideal body shape requires you to truly prove you want it by your actions.

Only the minority are willing to do what it takes. Only the minority are willing to make the required sacrifices. Only the minority are willing to endure the pain of that last rep when it feels impossible to complete it. Are you going to join the minority or stay as part of the majority? It is your choice.

As you start this journey you must be ready and willing to make all necessary sacrifices along the way. The better shape you are in to start with the less room for error there is. An individual who is obese or overweight will see results with the slightest changes in their lifestyle. But as they lose weight they will need to get stricter and make more sacrifices in order to continue to see progress. Once you have completed the initial 2-3 week phase of exercising your body will speed up it's adaptability ability. At this stage you must give 100% effort and intensity in training sessions to continue to experience fast results. It won't happen otherwise. You must put the effort in. Even if right now you are obese or very overweight you will have to put good effort in but just getting healthier and more active will yield results for a short while. Once you start seeing some plateau that is your indicator that you need to step it up. You will learn much more about the 3 Keys To Effective Training Programs In Chapter 6.

Be aware that even temporary moments of mental weakness will impact your results. Each training session will be a mental minefield as part of your mind will want to quit when going gets tough and the other part will want you to drive on and hit your full potential. Are you rethinking whether you are ready for this journey? Don't worry you are ready. Otherwise you wouldn't be reading this book right now. I just want to make sure that there are no misunderstandings about what it takes to get in shape. This is something that angers me about the majority of fitness and body transformation books. They sell you on the before and after pictures and give you a programme and give you the impression that it is just a case of following what the book says step by step. While this is true to a degree there needs to be much more clarity in what it takes mentally to achieve such a transformation as their success stories would share with you if you met them. The deciding factor is how strong you are mentally in each and every training session. It is easy to complete a workout and give it a good effort. However it is another story leaving absolutely nothing in the tank and knowing 100% hand on heart that there was nothing more you could have given to that workout. I want to highlight a key mindset shift that should help you to keep on track. See this journey as being your final journey. I promised you at the start of this book that it would be the last book you would need to read in this area. Get excited about this being your final transformation journey to your ideal body. You are going to achieve it and because you are doing it the right way maintenance will be easy once you get there.

The exciting news is that you are only weeks from your ideal body depending on your starting point. Even if you are months away you should be excited as it will be one final journey that will change your life forever. During your MSS journey you will create healthy mind/body/health habits that will serve you for life. In following this journey you are guaranteeing that you will never return to your former lifestyle and body shape.

MSS is designed for long term success not just short term. Once you follow the programme you will achieve super fast results but at the same time creating positive lifestyle habits. The one key question is – are you tough enough? Do you want this badly enough? You need to if you are going to make your goal a reality.

Your heart and soul needs to go into the next 6 weeks in particular. You will need to grit your teeth and push your pain barrier through the roof during training sessions. You will need to regularly get outside your comfort zone. Do you want to be in the best shape of your life or not? It is your choice.

Throughout the next 6 weeks you must remain laser focused and mentally strong as emphasised in section 1. I can't emphasise enough the importance of daily mindset training being a core part of your day, every single day. It will decide your level of success. You will need to smash through obstacles and challenges that life regularly throws at all of us. You must be ready to destroy excuses you will make along the way. You will need to become immune to discomfort, immune to temptation, immune to the opinions of others. This is your body. This is your life. Between now and the end of this book I will be giving you all the tools that you need to achieve your ideal body shape as well as in addition being in control of your mindset and health. You just need to apply them.

With my Metabolic Stimulation System programme you will stimulate your body like never before. In order to maximise this stimulation you will need to show determination and desire in every training session. Make sure you adhere to the MSS nutrition programme that compliments the MSS Exercise programme. You will witness results that will shock you. That will shock others. My strategies will turn you into a metabolic furnace, stripping fat at a rate you won't believe, sculpting and toning muscle to create a rock hard body. We start your journey focusing for just 6 weeks. Depending on your starting point this may be long enough or may be a massive kickstart to eventually achieving your ideal body shape goal after a few months.

The only question that remains to be asked a 3rd and final time is :

Are You Tough Enough?

How let's learn about effective exercise and destroy some myths.

2 – What Is Metabolism?

As I mentioned in the previous chapter getting lean and toned is determined by placing a focus on elevating both your basal and daily metabolic rate. Exercise is the most important factor in this. Do you understand what your basal and daily metabolic rates are? If not here are some definitions :

Basal Metabolic Rate is your personal level of calories that will be burned regardless of activity levels. These are the calories burned by your body to keep you alive and to allow the body's systems to deal with the basic demands placed on them.

Daily Metabolic Rate is the rate at which you will burn calories on a particular day which is impacted by your exercise and nutrition on that particular day.

Your Metabolism determines the rate at which you burn calories. Therefore positively impacting your metabolism is a crucial factor in achieving your ideal body shape. Your metabolic rate plays a key role in determining the speed at which you strip fat. Once you are maximising your potential to stimulate your metabolic rate via exercise you must then ensure that you adhere to an effective nutrition programme to create a calorie deficit while still feeding the body it's required nutrient level to function optimally. It is important that you do this in a healthy way with a long term lifestyle focus. This is not the case with the majority of diets. Hence why they usually yield only short term success with most reverting back to their pre diet shape if not worse. With MSS we will be creating a metabolic furnace which will both strip fat fast as well as ensuring that maintenance will be easy.

Simply put, the higher you elevate your metabolism, the more calories you will burn, the more fat you will lose and the quicker your results. When exercising it is so much more effective to focus on giving 100% to elevate your metabolism versus the typical measurements people focus on such as calories-burned, distance covered, duration etc. These figures will mean nothing if the required level of intensity was not applied. Also these measurements are not very accurate as usually just based on inputting your age and weight. Every single person has a different metabolic rate which is determined by age, activity levels and at that specific moment their metabolic rate is determined by what they have done previously that day. Intensity is the first of the 3 keys to achieving results which you will read more about these in Chapter 6 of this section. So focus on your intensity level and it's effect on your metabolism not what a calibrated machine tells you!

Let's go back to your basal metabolic rate. Your basal metabolic rate is effected by a number of factors :

- Your general levels of activity : more active = more calories burned at rest.
- Your level of fitness : fitter body = more calories burned at rest.

- Your muscle mass : more muscle mass = more calories burned at rest.
- Your age : each year from 25(on average) your metabolism slows down and you also lose muscle mass which decreases your calorie burning as muscle burns calories on ongoing basis throughout the day and night.

By living a healthy and active lifestyle, which includes both cardiovascular and resistance training, you will counteract the challenge of factor 4 above. Keep focused on factors 1 to 3. Make sense? Once you are conscious of your metabolism and focus on positively impacting it you not only start a journey to faster results but more importantly lifelong results. Positively impacting your metabolism is why the fitter, leaner and more sculpted you are the more difficult, if not impossible, it is to increase your bodyfat levels once you maintain a healthy active lifestyle. This is the exciting part as once you put in the hard work required for a short period of your life results are easy to maintain. Within 6 weeks on my MSS programme you will be burning hundreds more calories per day even while sitting down. It is for the reasons outlined in this paragraph that most gain fat and weight as they hit their 30s. They become generally less active. Become more sedentary. Their work (office based for most) and commuting (car, bus, tube, train) mainly involves sitting down. Training with weights becomes more sporadic so there is no counteraction to the natural muscle wastage. In addition to this decrease in metabolism and calorie burning, which is not counteracted, most consume more calories per day and much more junk calories as well as alcohol calories. So is it clear now why so many get out of shape fast? Including yourself?

Now let's focus on exercise's impact on your metabolism. There are 2 types of exercise that elevate your metabolism

- Cardiovascular training – elevates metabolism and burns calories from impact on heart and lungs
- Resistance training – body must repair muscle fiber damage and also maintain itself – this is a 24/7 process. Each pound of muscle burns anywhere from 10-50 calories depending on who you want to believe.

While doing cardio or resistance exercise will have an impact on your metabolism it is the level of workout intensity which is the key to getting the highest metabolic effect from both forms of exercise. Intensity will be covered in more depth in Chapter 6.

Intense cardiovascular exercise elevates your metabolism for a number of hours after exercise. Think about your time exercising as like revving the engine or winding up a toy. It is when you leave go that things really happen. The metabolic effect is dramatically higher with intense short duration cardio versus low to medium intensity steady state long duration cardio. Also intense exercise will positively impact your basal metabolic rate as you get fitter and gain more muscle mass while steady state exercise won't. The stimulation just isn't there with low to medium intensity steady state cardio. You will burn some calories during the workout but the post workout impact is minimal. Whereas with HIIT and Interval type training while the workout duration is much shorter the post workout impact lasts for hours. Think about it this way – In order to achieve anything in life that is worth achieving you must push your limits and get way outside your comfort zone to achieve progress and success. This principle applies to everything in life. I will explain all of this in more detail in chapter 6 in this exercise section.

I mentioned earlier that by including regular resistance training you will burn calories 24/7. This even includes while asleep. How? Here's how. The more lean muscle you have the more calories you burn as the body has to burn calories in the process of repairing the microfibre tears caused. This process continues while asleep. Also remember that the more muscle you have the more calories you are burning at rest as it impacts your basal metabolic rate. I mentioned earlier that you will burn between 10 to 50 calories more per pound of muscle mass added. It all depends on who you believe as to how many calories per pound. It is critical to include resistance training if you want to be lean and sculpted. It is impossible to achieve such a physique otherwise. However high intensity must be applied to each set for maximum results. This means reaching the point of muscle failure with each set. Without doing this the muscular stimulation will not occur and it will just be training vs progressive training. When you do resistance training you are looking to add lean muscle and benefit from the metabolic impact of this.

Your nutrition programme also impacts your metabolic rate. Each time you eat your digestive system has to kick into gear and go to work burning calories in the process. This will be explained in detail in section 3 which is dedicated to part 3 of our formula – Nutrition.

In summary you can elevate your metabolism by following effective exercise strategies. Following a correct nutrition plan will also maintain this elevated metabolic state. As you get fitter and gain lean muscle your basal metabolic rate will increase. If your metabolism is stimulated correctly you can burn calories 24/7 even while asleep.

3 – Why Ab Crunches Are A Waste Of Time

It was around October 1995, at the age of 17, when I finally gave in to the nagging and went to the gym with my friend Dave. As I shared in my story, at the start of this book, my impression of the gym environment was quite different to reality and I fell in love with this lifestyle. Not long after setting foot in the gym for the first time I started following specific body transformation type exercise routines both in the gym and at home. I had always been active as a kid and teenager playing various sports and generally playing around as kids do. This was long before the playstation and xbox so as kids we knew nothing else but being outside all day when not at school. When I commit to something I give it my all. I lived in the gym exercising up to 3-4 hours a day doing fitness classes, resistance training, using treadmills, ellipticals, stationary bikes and rowers. Spending time in the gym became my healthy obsession and became the place I felt happiest. I just loved the post workout feeling with the endorphin release and general feel good factor. I was determined to do whatever it took to achieve my goal of having a sixpack like the male models on the covers of the fitness and bodybuilding magazines I was reading.

I was willing to do whatever it would take to get a sixpack. Remember in earlier chapters I have stressed the importance of showing desire and determination. Without these traits any goal is unattainable and will just remain a dream and desire. I wanted results fast!! This meant that I was spending up to 3 hours training a day pushing my limits in pursuit of a lean muscular body and most importantly a sixpack. This was the prize I was after. I expected this to be the result once I put in the effort and showed the dedication. I read popular magazines, listened to the "hardcore" bodybuilders, attended fitness courses and seminars to gain the knowledge and then apply it. I attended as many exercise classes I could each week as well as my gym based exercise routine. The more you do the faster the results right?

Everything I was learning was pointing towards the need for 100s of crunches and various abdominal exercises on a daily basis. Being consistent and dedicated with this type of exercise was a necessity to get a sixpack. This made sense to me as I wanted to change how my abdominal area looked so naturally you must hammer that area. Right? You focus on the area you want to improve. You do as many exercises as you can for that area. Right? So I made a commitment to myself to complete a thousand repetitions of various abdominal exercises every single day hitting the abdominal area from every possible angle. Like with all my exercise and nutrition I was disciplined. I was consistent. I didn't dare miss a day. I was working my abs from all different angles, hitting the lower and upper abdominals as well as the obliques. I was spending up to 30 minutes a day specifically on working my abs. If I was serious about uncovering my abs and having a visible sixpack this was what was required so it had to be done. My overall workout plan included training time both at home and in the gym. This included aerobic classes (yes I was often the only guy with up to 120 women!! Had it's perks!), circuit training, running, rowing and resistance training on a daily basis. I was also following what was a strict nutrition plan for fat loss.

Now I want to fast forward to today. With extensive research and experimenting I no longer recommend any abdominal exercises when the goal is getting visible abs and a sixpack. What? Are you serious you are thinking. For over a decade now I rarely if ever do abdominal exercises myself. I rarely include them in client programmes. Without specifically targeting the abdominals with various crunch style exercises I manage to maintain a lean and toned midsection year round. This also applies to my clients who always question me early on when we start working together on the lack of abdominal focused exercises. They just can't understand how they are going to get visible abs without abdominal exercises but I am always proved right.

This is totally contradictory to what I shared in the previous paragraph regarding what I NEEDED to do in order to have visible abs. You would have expected that all of that effort and dedication I was putting in would have yielded a killer midsection, with chiselled abs right? You would be wrong. It didn't and even after months of discipline doing a thousand reps abdominal exercises daily I was no closer to having visible abs than I had been months previously. This was even after such intense abdominal focused sessions!!! But what about what all of the infomercials, magazines, books, the internet and even the courses I had invested in and attended tell us? They all promote and recommend lots of abdominal focused exercises to get visible abs. Were they lying and using deceitful marketing to make money? Are they misinformed? Outdated? Probably a mixture of all but I won't get into this subject now. The fact was that I and millions around the world were, and still are, being fed garbage. This is why through Metabolic Stimulation System I am committed to laying out the truth about not just getting in the best shape of your life but how to easily maintain it once you get there!! So let's get to the truth about what it takes to get abs.

Firstly let's review the regime I followed religiously on a daily basis. This regime was not only ineffective in giving me the results I wanted but disastrous physically in how I looked after a few months. The abdominal muscles are easily stimulated to grow. I was putting so much focused effort on this one area of my body that they grew quite substantially. Besides being stimulated, when you work them directly, your abdominals are also stimulated in most activities. For any multi joint, explosive or compound movement you need to keep a solid core area unless you are doing an isolated movement. These exercises stimulate and use the abdominal muscles. The squat exercise is actually the #1 exercise for the abdominals. Think about the pressure the whole core area is under when lowering and raising during this exercise. The core area will be recruited for all non machine based leg exercises. The core gives stability. Even when running or taking part in a circuit class you are working your abs even though not specifically targeting them. When you do boxing and kicking workouts you are engaging your core to maintain a stable base and to get power behind your punches and kicks. So the upshot of my months of dedicated ab work was that my abdominal wall grew significantly and naturally grew and pushed outwards. I now looked fatter not leaner as I had not actually lost any body fat around my midsection. That sure was a good return on my time/energy investment wouldn't you agree?

This section and the next section on nutrition are focused on going deep into exercise and nutrition strategies so that you fully understand what works and why and as a result you are more likely to stick to the program. These two sections contain the key secrets to getting lean, toned and achieving visible abs. I don't want you to experience the many years of frustration I did. MSS is designed to fast track your success by me sharing everything I now know that I would follow if I was to go back in a time machine. The most frustrating part of that period of my life was that despite the hours of daily exercise i was doing in combination with what I believed was a healthy fat loss nutrition programme there was only minimal difference in the leanness and definition of my midsection area. For sure my fat levels had decreased all over my body and I had gained lean muscle and didn't look too bad but my goal remained having visible abs.

When I used to check myself out, sideways view, in the mirror my abdominals were actually ahead of my chest. This should be the other way around!! If I had been super lean and ripped this wouldn't have been a big deal but I wasn't. The layer of fat on my stomach area was more or less the same as it had been months before. My abdominal muscles were just bigger making me look worse in my opinion. As a result of minimal fat loss and growing abdominal muscles I now looked fatter – how soul destroying do you think that was? I was so disillusioned and angry. I had read loads of books, completed many courses, spoken to many "expert" trainers yet my results were minimal. What was going on? It was time to discover the truth about achieving visible abs and lowering bodyfat levels. It was time for extensive research and to find solutions.

Here is the truth about revealing visible abs. My next statement is going to shock and surprise you.

You already have a sixpack

We all do. You have a skeleton and on this skeleton are your muscles and then we all vary in the level of fat we have on our muscles. This is who all of our bodies consist of. However the visibility of your muscles depends on your bodyfat level. The lower this is the more visible your muscles including your abdominals. When you work your muscles they become harder and even grow depending on what type of routine you are following but we all have muscles. I want to add here too that it is impossible for muscle to turn to fat or vice versa as is often said about inactive people. They are totally different and unique substances. It is like saying a chair turned into water. When you don't use muscle it gets soft and saggy with the texture of fat but it is still muscle. And you either lose or gain muscle or fat. One cannot convert to the other – make sense? If we didn't our bodies would not function and move correctly. Does that make sense?

Solely completing abdominal crunches is not how you reveal abs. Abdominal exercises will not shift the layer of abdominal fat that covers them. They will just work and develop the abdominal muscles. Your goal is to burn fat and the more fat your burn the lower your body fat percentage which in turn will result in visible abs once you reach a bodyfat level of 10% and under for a guy and 20% and under for a female. How do we increase our fat burning potential? Raise your basal and daily metabolic rate as we spoke of in the previous chapter. Is it starting to make more sense now? Are you starting to see why you have been fighting a losing battle up to now?

I want to take this opportunity to clarify something. Most don't realise this but you are actually working your abdominals throughout each and every day. And I am referring to non exercise or home based exercise. Just normal day to day movements. You recruit your abdominal muscle fibres every time you sit up straight at your desk, while you are driving, each time you stand back up off the toilet or the couch or step out of a car. Every time you move your body or reach you are using your abdominals. You naturally and unconsciously contract the core area when moving or you wouldn't be able to do such simple tasks. Each time you exercise whether running up a hill or using the rower or throwing a punch you recruit abdominal muscle fibres. Every time you lift something off the ground or reach up for something you recruit abdominal muscle fibres. The fact is that many movements in our daily lives recruit the abdominals as you must contract them in order to protect your spinal column. You do this naturally. The abdominals work in combination with the erector spinae (lower back) muscle to protect your spinal column. This area around your midsection is what is referred to as the core area.

As I mentioned earlier in this chapter the squat exercise is the single most effective abdominal exercise you can do, recruiting more abdominal fibres than any other exercise. Think about the work your core does during this movement. Any loaded bodyweight exercise where you must support yourself, holding a stable position throughout the movement results in core contractions to protect the spine while working your abdominals. Now of course this assumes correct technique is being followed but this should always be the case.

The "ab solution" as I will refer to it is a billion if not trillion dollar industry. Each year we are bombarded with adverts and infomercials featuring the latest ab device, diets, fat burners and vibration belts. All marketing is focused on getting visible abs. People are buying into the false hope that it can be this easy. Manufacturers are not going to tell you the truth as they are focused on making profit. There is no money in healthy fit looking people. Only in those who dream of being so. All of these "ab solutions" are a complete waste of time, energy and money. As I stressed in the previous chapter your focus needs to be on positively impacting your metabolism through exercise and nutrition and also on creating a healthy active lifestyle.

Raising your metabolism through intense structured training regimes is what will melt that layer of fat over your abdominals not crunches or gimmicks. In addition to this your nutrition plan plays a key role as you will learn in Section 3. You can't exercise yourself out of a poor diet. And it's not about focusing on how many calories you ingest daily but rather the type of calories and the timings. More about this in Section 3. For over a decade I have rarely allocated time for ab exercises. Even when I was in the best shape of my life, winning the 'Body For Life' competition in 2004, with chiselled abs and only 5% bodyfat, I rarely included abs in my gruelling regime training twice a day one hour at a time at maximum intensity. Abdominal work was a tiny percentage of my overall training programme and was incorporated more for final shaping of the abdominal region versus as part of the journey to lowering bodyfat levels in achieving visible abs.

Don't get me wrong – there is a certain benefit to abdominal work particularly when there may be muscular imbalances or lower back issues and for improving athletic performance. However what I am focused on sharing in this book is body transformation. My main point is that if you are going to allocate any time to abdominal exercises never do so at the sacrifice of time you should be spending on cardio and resistance training. These modes of exercise are what stimulate your metabolism, burn fat and build lean muscle. Metabolic Stimulation is the key to elevating your metabolism and peeling away that stubborn layer of abdominal fat.

In summary my message to you in this chapter is to quit wasting time on your abdominal exercises and classes. Start focusing on metabolism boosting cardio and resistance training. What are the most effective metabolic stimulating types of cardio and resistance training? I will explain in the next two chapters. In the next chapter I will explain why steady state low intensity cardio will make you fatter not leaner! You are probably shocked by this statement too lol.

4 – Why Steady State Low Intensity Cardio Is Useless and Makes You Fat

In this chapter I want to educate you on why low intensity steady state cardio is useless and a waste of your time and energy. I do want to make sure however that you are clear that this statement refers to situations when your goal is to lose body fat and achieve a body transformation where you are in your ideal body shape. Steady state cardio has a big role to play in endurance sports (in addition to HIIT and Interval type workouts) such as triathlon which I compete in. And also LISS cardio is great for general health and wellbeing and releasing endorphins. But LISS Cardio is ineffective for losing fat so you have visible abs and has no positive effect on gaining lean muscle whereas HIIT actually does.

What I am also including in this type of training is heart training zone focused workouts. Supposedly you should workout at 60-70% of your max heart rate (220 minus your age) to optimise fat burning. This type of training protocol is taught in all fitness courses. There are also stickers on machines and charts in gyms giving instructions and outlining the benefits for fat burning. This type of training protocol is totally ineffective and makes even less sense the older you are as you are working at such a low heart rate. It takes no account of different fitness levels which would have a big bearing on how hard a certain heart rate will feel. For example if I am pushing to my absolute maximum I would be hitting about 150-160 BPM tops. However if you are totally unfit and out of condition you would probably feel medium intensity at this same heart rate range and your maximum would be more likely be the 190-200 range. So this protocol takes no account of individual situations and overall is totally ineffective anyway. It is true that you are going to be burning just fat at such low intensity as it won't trigger the body to use glycogen stores BUT the level of fat calories burned will be at such a low level it will be insignificant. Also again I will go back to something I mentioned a few times in the last chapter. Anything worth achieving in life takes a lot of effort and getting outside your comfort zone. While no one likes being on a treadmill for an hour the fact remains that if you are following 60-70% heart training zone or just doing steady state low intensity exercise it is not difficult and is just boring. So how can it possibly stimulate your body enough to force change? It is just common sense!

The focus in every one of your workouts should be revving the engine so that you are burning the maximum amount of calories post workout and in general via raising your basal metabolic rate. Personally my belief is that this whole LISS heart training zone protocols are there more for safety in a gym environment and also in the belief that if exercise feels easy (while boring as hell) more may do it. Those who recommend such training methods may believe or hope this will occur but it is not the case. There is also what many would consider conspiracy theory that top industries including the health/wellbeing/fitness industry does not want to see people getting results as there is no money in healthy people. Make of that what you want.

When I first qualified over 20 years ago heart training zone cardio workouts were what I had been taught to be the most effective. Naturally I followed this protocol as if I learned it in the course it had to be the most effective. However with every client they would hit a plateau after following this LISS heart training zone protocol for a period of time. And this was only with those who would be considered obese or very overweight. Those I worked with who were in decent shape saw minimal results. Thankfully I was doing some resistance training with them so they saw some! Regular exercisers experienced very little benefit from such workouts in terms of both fitness and body fat loss.

I took pride in my reputation and wanted the best for my clients. And remember I wanted to be the best too. My goal was to become #1 from the very start as I shared at the start of this book. This is why I began extensive research into new training methods as I wanted my clients to achieve the fastest results. Results are all that count in this industry and when people are not seeing results they lose motivation, blame their trainer, give up and look for another trainer, training method or diet. I have always wanted my clients to achieve fast but more importantly lasting lifelong results. Being on the right exercise programme is key to this but also is the element of education. This is why I put such a huge focus on explaining the WHY of everything I tell you and anyone I work with.

Let me continue by once again explaining why I can make such a statement as I have about LISS cardio being "useless". In doing so I am questioning you and other practitioners of this type of training.. To achieve anything in life you must get outside your comfort zone and do what makes you uncomfortable. You must push your boundaries and perceived limitations. The same principle applies to all areas of life.

The question I have for you then is – why do most exercisers not realise that it is impossible to get lean and toned by following a low intensity steady state heart training zone type cardio workout? Do they just hope it works? Are they not willing to do the logical thing and work harder and just be happy to have an excuse that they are following the programme/advice which must be the problem not them? Or are most people just so damn confused and lead astray by the industry and "experts" that they have no idea what they should do? I presume you are one of these people so which is it? Ask yourself these questions. How can one lose bodyfat and get lean when no real pressure and stimulation is being applied to the body? When no limits are being pushed? LISS heart training zone workouts are just long duration and only challenging mentally in combating the boredom factor so mentally challenging more than physically. Why would getting in shape be so much different than the level of sacrifice, effort and desire required to say gaining a promotion or generating a million dollars in 12 months? To achieve anything in life you must push your limits. Does this make sense?

If you are not experiencing an intense cardio workout then you are not creating the required metabolic stimulation that is required for change. Cardio HIIT (High Intensity Interval Training) is the only effective fat burning cardio to follow. It can also be called interval training or tabata but more or less the same principles applied under different name. During such workouts you must push your limits during a short duration like 15 to 60 seconds and then follow with recovery time which can be anything from 30 seconds to 3 or 4 minutes depending on your fitness and recovery levels. By putting your body under these phases of high intensity you are stimulating your metabolism and revving the engine like I describe it as. With LISS and heart training zone workouts the focus is on calories being burned during the workout but this is the totally wrong approach. What you need to be more concerned about is how many calories you can burn post workout and in general via your basal metabolic rate (calorie burning at rest). So with HIIT training you are revving the engine during the workout and then post workout your metabolism really takes off raising to a very high level. Your calorie burning (metabolic rate) will be seriously high for a few hours post workout. Also if you have pushed your body to it's limit you will increase your fitness levels each workout and this will increase your basal metabolic rate too. This means that in a month's time you will be burning hundreds more calories while sitting down versus this moment if you apply the MSS exercise programme principles. Sound good? I hope all this is making sense. I am doing my best to explain it in as simple a way as I can. I want you to understand WHY HIIT is the only way to train for cardio when the goal is to strip fat fast and lose belly fat in particular.

In the title of this chapter I mentioned that LISS makes you fat. I am sure this would have shocked you just like saying that LISS is useless. So let me explain why I made this statement so you can understand why I said it. Now the title is a little misleading if you read it directly as "steady state makes you fat" and it meaning straight away if you follow it. I expect most will read it this way. What does happen is that prolonged periods of following a steady state low intensity cardio programme will contribute to other factors which in combination will increase fat storage and make it more difficult to lose fat. If the wrong conditions are in place your body will easily store fat and find it difficult to use fat as fuel. Steady state cardio completed over a long period of time actually promotes fat storage. Not only does your fat burning gene and hormones switch off but from 25 years on your metabolism actually slows down annually and without boosting your metabolism through intense exercise your calorie surplus increases resulting in increases in bodyfat levels. Have you noticed that many gym goers or road walkers actually get fatter over time not slimmer? You may have even noticed this trend in your own body. If you are not training to get fitter then you are not counteracting this natural metabolic decrease. And for this reason you are going to gain fat. Make sense now?

So from now on ditch the low intensity steady state cardio routines and instead follow HIIT workout and cardio interval training. Then you will start experiencing rapid fat loss.

The cardio part of your MSS programme involves interval training and high intensity mini circuits. Once again I repeat do not waste your time with steady state cardio or following heart training zones. I would expect after reading this chapter you never will again. I hope so. HIIT will see your metabolism elevating for hours afterwards and is the fastest way of stripping fat. Remember if you force your body out of it's comfort zone it adapts so you have the ability to create new limits each and every training session. If at the end of each HIIT session you can honestly say you gave it your best for each interval you have done what you needed to do. Be honest with yourself as only fooling yourself otherwise!!

In the next chapter I am going to educate you on the #1 method to creating a metabolic furnace so you can maximise your fat burning.

5 – The Key To Creating A Metabolic Furnace

After reading the previous chapter I hope you now clearly understand why steady state low intensity cardio is a waste of time when aiming to transform your body shape. When you are obese or totally inactive it will yield results initially but this will slow down and eventually plateau. The benefits will become more from a health perspective. Taking care of one's health is so important but in this book we are focused on what will transform your body and burn the most bodyfat. If I was to ask you which of cardio and resistance training is the fastest way to burn fat what would your answer be? The majority would answer cardio but they would be totally wrong. Were you? Contrary to popular belief resistance training is the #1 exercise mode for stripping fat and getting lean and toned. Consistently following a resistance training programme creates a metabolic furnace that burns calories 24/7 even while asleep! Let me explain why.

Do you believe that all of these Hollywood stars, international popstars, athletes and models have achieved their physiques from just cardio? Do you think Jennifer Aniston got her sought after toned arms from cardio alone? This is actually impossible. Without resistance training such lean toned physiques are impossible.

Effective cardio exercise, as outlined in the last chapter, yields many benefits and should be included as an important part of any body transformation programme. However if you exclude resistance training from the overall workout plan you will never ever get lean enough for visible abs and it will be impossible to get tight and toned with defined lean muscle.

Why is resistance training so important? There are many reasons. The more lean muscle you have the higher your basal metabolic rate and from the age of 25 onwards you should be aiming to counteract the muscle wasting process that occurs naturally for everyone as I have previously mentioned. Therefore you need to follow a resistance training programme to counteract this natural metabolic drop. If you are female don't worry as this does not mean you have to build big bulky muscles. Whether male or female our focus is on building lean muscle not size. Men will naturally build some size with weight training due to higher testosterone levels but a female could do the same program exactly and won't gain size. Resistance training also positively impacts your metabolic rate throughout the day. When you consistently follow a resistance training programme your basal metabolic rate elevates. This means that you are burning more calories at rest.

With Resistance training calorie burning occurs 24/7 as your body is in a constant state of repair. Your workouts create microfibre tears which nutrition and rest then repair but during this process you are burning loads of calories. Even better news is that with resistance training you even burn calories while you sleep as this is when the majority of the repair process will take place.

Are you more enthused and eager to lift weights now? Another major benefit, especially for females, is that it is the best way to increase bone density. Resistance training on a regular basis will dramatically cut your bone age so focus on that versus what the media tell you about needing to consume dairy products and take medications to protect bones. I'll get into these lies in the nutrition section.

By following the MSS programme your metabolism will be dramatically faster in just 6 weeks. However so many people regularly follow resistance training programmes but with little results apart from a little bit of toning up and getting a bit stronger. Why is this? It is for this reason that digesting and implementing what I teach you in the next chapter is going to be so crucial to your results. Without applying the 3 keys I outline in that chapter your results will be minimal, zero or even negative! I have mentioned a few times about how important intensity is and this is no different with resistance training. You must annihilate your body ripping your muscle fibres apart (I know it sounds terrible but it is good) in each resistance training session. You must push your limits so that you couldn't complete even one more repetition in any set. In each set you need to reach the point of muscular failure (inability to complete another repetition). If you have a training partner or personal trainer you can even go beyond this point using negatives, eccentrics, assisted reps, isometric etc. There is no benefit to sub-maximum sets in your workout, except for your warm up sets. I want to remind you again that your goal when training is the stimulation of your muscles and this will only happen if they are pushed to the point of muscular failure. Remember if it was a case of just doing some weights everyone would look lean and toned. If you look around any gym there are not many that are. Getting in shape takes consistent work and is far from easy. If there is anyone in the gym who appears to never push themselves yet look fantastic it is likely this is down to either steroids or incredible genetics and metabolism. Next you need to know what the most effective form of resistance training is for fat burning, getting lean and sculpted.

In the MSS programme you will be following a Peripheral Heart Action style workout for your resistance training workouts. Peripheral Heart Action involves completing a series of compound exercises consecutively while alternating between upper and lower body exercises. This strategy elevates your metabolism to a very high level as your body must transport blood to the muscles being used. It makes an anaerobic activity very aerobic. When working the lower body the body must send blood to the leg muscles. Then when you switch to an upper body exercise the body must then work hard to send blood up to those muscles from the legs. So this is creating an aerobic effect in combination with the anaerobic activity that is happening via resistance training. This style of resistance training is very intense from a muscle stimulation point of view but also pushes the heart and lungs which is what creates such a great overall metabolic effect.

Like all aspects of the MSS programme the resistance training is focused on short intense bouts of exercise followed by rest. During your MSS resistance training programme you will work intensively for about one minute per exercise in a ten exercise circuit and will take just 15-30 seconds recovery between exercises. It is important you stick to the recovery period rigidly as it is important to the aerobic aspect of the workout. Then take 2 minutes rest between circuits. Each circuit will last about 15 minutes and you can complete up to 3 circuits depending on the time you have available.

It is very important that for each repetition of any exercise you :

1. Complete the repetition with full range of motion. This means that you fully stretch and contract the muscle. So complete the exercise going the full range of movement that the muscle and joint will allow.
2. Adhere to a TUT (Time Under Tension) Of 4021 – this means that for the eccentric/negative phase you do a 4 count, then pause for 1 second, contraction phase over 2 seconds and start eccentric phase with 0 second rest. Make sure to count seconds as 1, 1000 vs just 1. When you count just numbers they won't be real seconds. Remember this TUT is very important especially the eccentric phase of 4 seconds as this is where the most microfibre tears are made and this is the most crucial part of every repetition.
3. Only work the muscles are you meant to be working. So make sure you keep the right technique and the only movement should be of the muscles you are aiming to recruit. Resist the temptation to "cheat" by swinging and decreasing the range of movement. If you can't do a repetition right don't do it.
4. Breath out on exertion. Do your best to breath out on the contraction phase and in on the eccentric phase. Otherwise you are a lot of internal pressure and

raising blood pressure. I do appreciate that when you are getting close to the point of muscular failure it can be difficult to avoid holding your breath. Keep to the breathing plan as long as you can.

For the purpose of repetition if you want to achieve a lean sculpted body your body must be pushed to its absolute limit. Ask yourself after your workout – could I have given another ounce of energy to that workout? Could I have completed even one more repetition with controlled technique? Could I have been more controlled during time under tension? If your answers are no then that's a job well done and you are a step closer to achieve your best body.

6 – The 3 Keys To Effective Training Programmes

Throughout this book I have mentioned Intensity quite a few times and have repeatedly stressed how important it is as one of the 3 key factors to effective exercise and results. Without applying intensity you will achieve little results from your exercise efforts. Without applying the other 2 key factors you also have little chance of achieving any significant results. Your goal with exercise is metabolic and muscular stimulation. The next step is repairing the muscle fibres post workout through good nutrition and rest. Without each of these being in place results once again are impossible. I want to stress to you that getting results is so much more scientific than just doing more exercise and eating healthier. That is a myth. I will be educating you on everything you need to know about nutrition and what an effective nutrition plan is in the next section and then sleep strategies in section 4. But right now let's focus on what these 3 keys to effective exercise are.

Here is the reality :

You could spend (and you may already) two hours per day, six days per week working out at home or in the gym for the next twenty years and experience minimal results. I know this may defy logic for you but it is fact. This will be even more likely if you are already in good shape and just looking to lose a few more % body fat to gain visible abs or looking to gain a few more pounds of lean muscle.

If you are someone who trains regularly have you been feeling for a while that you have reached a plateau? Have you found it near impossible to experience further fat loss despite your best efforts? On the other hand if you have not exercised consistently for a while or are a yo yo dieter I want you to think back to a time when you got results from exercise. Did you find that previously when you started exercising consistently you experienced results but then they just stopped after a while even though you changed nothing? You reached this plateau even though you continued to put the same effort in as you had been when you experienced results? It doesn't make sense right? These experiences are common and, from my point of view, to be expected for the majority of people who exercise regularly or sporadically. However you must realise that this is valuable feedback. It is feedback that you are doing something wrong as otherwise it would be working. Right? Let me explain why what you have been doing has not been working. Then I will share the 3 keys to effective training and lasting results.

If like most you have spent years focusing on quantity when it comes to exercising then this is one of the main reasons why you have not achieved the results you would have expected from your efforts. Remember I shared earlier in the book that I used to exercise up to 3 hours a day 6 days a week and with minimal results. Your need to shift your mindset and focus to quality over quantity. This is where the 3 keys come in. Most people believe that they need to exercise for a minimum of an hour minimum for it to be effective. Some even exercise daily for 90 to 120 minutes or more. The ironic thing is, that by exercising for so long you are guaranteeing that it will be a waste of time (I want to stress again that this viewpoint is from a body transformation point of view as all exercise is good for health).

You may believe that during this session you were exercising intensively but the fact that you are still not in your ideal body shape is proof otherwise. Also importantly it is impossible to exercise at maximum intensity for such a long duration of time. The most anyone can exercise intensively for is about 45 minutes as after this time you won't be able for more, both mentally and physically, if the workout has been intense enough. So your workouts have not been intense enough and possibly weren't even effective enough in their initial design. There is no way one can focus and give 100% for 90 mins to 2 hours. The only you can exercise intensively for such a long period of time is if there are loads of breaks during the workout. This is typical on the gym floor with most spending more time talking versus exercising. Sticking to prescribed rest periods is key to the whole routine and this is why long breaks talking are decreasing the overall effectiveness of the workout.

By implementing the MSS principles you will have better results exercising even just 15 minutes a few days a week compared to those who spend up to 2 hours exercising 6 days a week. Quality not quantity is what gets results.

I want to make sure you fully understand how ineffective low to medium intensity long duration exercise is. I addressed this in the cardio chapter and to a degree in the resistance chapter but let me stress this point again as it can never be stressed enough. Your body is an amazing machine and is designed to adapt to whatever challenges and stimulation is put on it. When you exercise at low to medium intensity your body – muscles, lungs, heart – has no problem coping with the pressure being applied as this challenge was met before and the body is more than capable of dealing with it. Of course some days you may be mentally weaker or less focused so such workouts feel more challenging mentally but physically they are not. This is why many recreational endurance athletes are never lean and may even be overweight. They are not giving their body any reason to burn excess fat. They are not stimulating the metabolism. Whereas when you push your body to it's limits it must and will adapt and strengthen itself ready for the next challenge. This adaptation phase results in high calorie burning. Once you then follow a sensible balanced nutrition plan your body will renew itself stronger, fitter and leaner ready for the next challenge. At the end of each workout the only question you need to ask yourself is – could I have given more? If you answer no then job done.

So the first of the 3 keys to getting lean is stimulation through intensity once it is applied to an effective training programme and combined with a sensible balanced nutrition plan. When you get fitter your basal metabolism increases. If you add lean muscle your metabolism will increase as will your daily calorie burning. You need to push far beyond your normal pain threshold. Whatever you feel your limit has been, believe me you can go beyond that. You reading this book proves that intensity likely hasn't been applied to the right level as if you were in your ideal body shape you wouldn't be reading this right? You should finish your workout knowing that you could not have given another ounce of effort. You maxed out on everything whether HIIT cardio or PHA resistance.

During my victorious 'Body For Life Challenge' training regime I used to be on my knees gasping for air after just a 15-minute interval session. The high intensity phases in this workout only amounted to 5 minutes in total but each interval was given 100%. I was annihilating my body, which resulted in the stimulation required to drive my metabolism through the roof. During resistance training I was often screaming as my pain threshold was tested. My resistance training regime involved reaching failure followed by 3 assisted repetitions, followed by 3 eccentric repetitions and then supersetted with another exercise for the same muscle group with the same crushing intensity methods applied. It was torture but it was necessary to achieve my goal. I was pushing way beyond muscular failure point (in terms of reps that could be completed full range of motion unassisted). The more levels of intensity you apply the more muscle fibre damage is created. Remember your goal in each workout is to rip as much muscle fibres as possible.

So focus on intensity, intensity, intensity. Intensity creates the stimulation required for fast results. So that is Key #1. Onto Key #2 – Progression.

Your body is truly amazing. There is actually no limit to what can be achieved physically. This applies to your fat and lean muscle levels and overall body shape or in athletic performance. This is why world records are always broken and why one can have visible abs even in their 70s and 80s. Once the right stimulation and strategies are being applied consistently this will result. So the second key is progression. In order to create your ideal body shape you must ensure that you progress or at least aim to progress each and every workout. No two workouts should ever be the same. The human body has no limits as I have said and has incredible ability to adapt to stimulation. So in every workout aim to do more than the previous one. What I recommend clients to do (and do myself) is to plan the next workout during their workout. This way you know exactly how you are feeling at that moment and can effectively plan for progress in the next workout. So for example if I did cardio and I did a HIIT session of 60 seconds at 6.0 mph and then 30 seconds at 9.0mph I would note to aim for at least 2 to 5 intervals of 6.0mph vs 9.2mph for the next workout. If it was resistance and I did 10 reps of 30 kg on an exercise I would note to aim for either 12 reps at 30 kg or 8 or 10 reps of 35 kg on the next workout. Always aim for progress no matter how small it may be. Depending on how you feel and how focused you are at the time you should hit your targets each time or close enough. But the main thing is to aim for progress. A bad night's sleep, stress or poor pre workout nutritional choices could effect performance but always plan for progress. So the first 2 keys are intensity and progression. When applied together these create fast results.

Now for the 3rd key to fast lasting results. It is muscle confusion. Although you may be applying intensity and progression it is not guaranteed that you will continue to lose fat and gain lean muscle over a period of time. Without muscle confusion you will notice a decrease or plateau in your results within 2 to 4 weeks on a programme. The scary thing is that most who get programmes, in a gym or from terrible unknowledgable or disinterested PTs, are on the same programme for months and often even for a whole year!! After 2 weeks that programme became less effective and after 4 to 6 weeks became ineffective. It doesn't matter how hard you were working out or how good your nutrition was during this time. When you start a new programme you experience great progress once the first 2 keys are applied. However even with applying the first 2 keys results slow down and a plateau is reached somewhere between 2 and 4 weeks on a programme. Your body gets bored and becomes unstimulated and you also get bored mentally. We as humans are wired for stimulation and new challenges. Often once 4 weeks have passed you end up going through the motions. Lack of results is a big demotivator. So it is between 2 to 4 weeks where muscle confusion plays an important role. From my experience you should change your routine every 2 weeks.

When I work with clients who need seriously fast results in a very short period of time – like for a wedding or holiday or shoot in 2 weeks – we change the routine every single workout. The Metabolic Stimulation System programme implements this strategy as I want you to experience the fastest results possible in the next 6 weeks.

This way you keep your body guessing all the time. You keep it stimulated. You are also mentally stimulated by this constant change and new challenge. The change can be in the exercises for particular muscles, order of exercises in a particular routine, TUT, number of reps, number of sets, HIIT recovery/hard ratio, number of intervals etc. Are you getting the idea?

So to summarise this chapter there are 3 keys to fast lasting results :

1. Intensity
2. Progression
3. Muscle confusion

Implement all 3 in tandem and you will experience incredible results in just weeks. I hope at this stage you can clearly understand why what you have been doing up to this point regarding exercise has been ineffective and yielded little results. I hope also that now you can understand why my strategies work so well and has seen thousands of my clients achieve incredible transformations in just weeks.

Now it is your turn.

Over the last 6 chapters we have covered the theoretical part of Exercise. Now it is time to outline what the Metabolic Stimulation System Exercise programme is in the next chapter.

7 – *Your 6-Week MSS Exercise Programme*

I hope by now that I have extensively and adequately explained the theoretical side of exercise. Now it is time to explain the MSS Exercise programme which you will follow for the next 6 weeks and beyond. In the last chapter I explained the 3 key effective training strategies that must be implemented for maximum results. In section 1 of this book I explained the importance of mindset and committing to a daily mental training programme which I also outlined for you. Your job now is to implement these strategies while following the MSS exercise programme. I am really excited for you as I know the results and changes that lie ahead for you. I know 100% that you and everyone around you will be shocked by the results you will experience in just the next few weeks.

Firstly before I talk you through the layout of the exercise programme I must stress the importance of measuring, tracking and analysing your progress on a weekly basis. I have provided a MSS progress chart in the resources section for you to track your progress. I want you to take certain measurements which I will outline shortly. Step 1 is to record your starting statistics and also set your target finishing stats. Your goal statement from section 1 should cover this. Next I want you to commit to taking your measurements at the end of each week so we can track and monitor your progress. This will ensure that you are moving at the desired pace to achieve your goal. Your progress chart will allow you to review and analyse progress and tweak anything where necessary. Your level of progress is going to be a direct result of how well you adhere to your training and nutrition programme. You can download your MSS progress chart at the resources link you can find at the back of this book.

Remember that you must apply the 3 keys to effective exercise in every workout to get the most from your training sessions. There is no time to lose so make every second count. The 3rd key muscle confusion is already incorporated into the programme so you must focus on implementing the other 2 keys which you have control over – intensity and progression. With MSS you have the opportunity to achieve faster results than anything you have experienced before with the added bonus of results being easily maintained after the 6 weeks. What will prove crucial is winning the daily mental battle. The lazy guy//girl in your head will do everything in his/her power to stop you taking action.

While I have included a space for tracking your weight on the MSS progress chart I must stress that it is more important that you track your bodyfat % and tape measurements rather than your weight. I am not a fan of tracking weight and I haven't weighed clients in about 15 years. I included weight on the MSS progress chart because many will want to track weight no matter what I say. Conditioning is hard to break. Here is why I hate weighing oneself as a progress tracker. Your weight is dependent on many factors outside of your control. Your weight is your weight at that precise moment in time. Even just 1 hour later it is highly likely to be different just as it would have been an hour before. This is even without exercising or eating during that hour.

If I were to hold you into a room for 24 hours and took your weight every hour it would likely be different every hour. This would be despite the fact that during that time there is nothing you would have done to improve or disimprove your body shape and fat levels. But the weight will have changed as internally the body is working away 24/7. For females a reliance on weight is a nightmare as 3 weeks out of every 4 their weight will be erratic due to hormones and time of the month(week before, during and after). For everyone your bowel movements and level of hydration will have a big impact on your weight at a particular moment. You might weigh yourself and then 30 minutes need to go to the toilet. This will effect your weight. Is this making sense? If you are still determined to track your weight then please use it only as a guide. Don't be too dependent on it. Take more notice of your bodyfat %, tape measurements, clothes and also your photos which I will get to later. These are reliable and real progress indicators as they will reflect whether you are actually changing or not. They are either improving or not. No factor impacts them apart from clothes very slightly if bloated.

Bodyfat measures the % of actual fat on your body. Once taken correctly this is a very accurate measurement. Focus on improving your fat levels as it is actually fat you want to lose not weight. If the scales were to decrease but your body shape and fat levels didn't would you be happy? Of course not. All you really care about is your fat levels and how well you fit into your clothes. So please use such indicators instead of the weighing scales. The most accurate method of measuring body fat apart from underwater weighing is using a skinfold callipers. Either get a trained professional at your gym to take your measurement or you can purchase a callipers yourself and learn how to use it. The most important thing is that the same person takes the measurements each week to ensure consistency and accuracy. Take measurements at the following points :

- Vertical measurement at midway point at front of upper arm (bicep)
- Vertical measurement at midway point at back of upper arm (tricep)
- Diagonal measurement at right shoulder blade (subscapular)
- Diagonal measurement at right hip bone (suprailiac)

Take each of these measurements on the RHS of your body. You then use a body fat chart to work out the % body fat.

Each week also take your tape measurements in the following areas :

- Circumference around mid chest and upper back
- Circumference around waist starting at belly button level
- Circumference around widest part of hips (If female)
- Midway point of upper arm (both arms)
- Midway point of upper thigh (both arms)

You can also take measurements in other areas such as neck and calves if you wish.

I also want you to use your clothes as a progress tracker. Are they fitting better in certain areas of overall? Are you fitting into a smaller size? I also want you to select an item of clothing you want to be able to wear comfortably once you reach your desired outcome. Try this on every few weeks to monitor and gauge how close you are getting.

The final progress tracker I want you to use is weekly photos. These are powerful tools not just for tracking progress but staying motivated too. Take a starting photo in your bikini/swimsuit(female) or shorts(male) with a front, side and back view. Then take photos at the end of each week. When you look at yourself in the mirror your state of mind has a big impact on what you see. Your view of yourself is determined by your mood at that moment. Sometimes you will think you look fantastic and see progress and other times you will think you look fat, out of shape and showing no visible sign of progress. However with a photo what you see is reality as you can't alter in your mind what the photo is showing you. This is why it is such a powerful progress tracking tool. Make sense?

I designed the MSS Exercise programme with the expectation that you will complete 6 training days per week, for the duration of the next 6 weeks, with 1 training session per day. As you are reading this I am assuming that you are serious about achieving fast results. Committing to 6 days training per week for the 6 weeks will yield maximum results. However if you only feel comfortable committing to 3 or 4 training sessions a week that is fine. However remember I have designed the programme in such a way that your workout can be

15mins, 30mins or 45 mins so that there should be no excuses for anyone not fitting in their exercise daily. The most important thing is consistency and creating a daily routine. I would urge you to make sacrifices and prioritise time for the MSS exercise programme for the next 6 weeks. Give it the time and you will experience the results. Like anything you get out of something what you put into it.

On monday, wednesday and friday, you will complete a cardiovascular workout. On tuesdays, thursdays and saturdays it will be resistance training. It is important that you stick to the programme layout as it is designed as it is so that you achieve maximum results. I recommend that you train first thing each morning where possible. This will achieve the best results. Training first thing in the morning is the most effective time to train as your only energy source is fat so you maximise fat burning. Also you elevate your metabolic rate from the start of the day and you can maintain this higher metabolic rate throughout the day once you adhere to your nutrition programme. Be willing to make whatever sacrifices you must to exercise first thing in the morning– it is only for 6 weeks. However if this is not suitable with your lifestyle and commitments don't worry. Just make sure to make time for the workout at some other stage that day. Also as I outline in the nutrition section exercise up to 3 hours after a meal to allow the food to digest and also be burned as fuel during this time. This way you are increasing your chances of exercising in a fasted state similar to when exercising first thing in the morning. At worst you will start with much depleted glycogen stores in your muscles so you will move to burning fat as your fuel early into the workout.

You must take one rest day each week. This is very important as you will need to recharge both mentally and physically. It is not good for anyone to train 7 days a week. You will be working at a high intensity level every workout and you need to be focused and alert every workout. Put all your mental and physical energy into the other 6 days and switch off for your rest day. It should feel needed.

Your programme involves completing one intense training session each day. Should there be occasions where you would like to fit in an extra training session (just in case you ever get urge to) use the following guidelines:

Resistance training days :

15 minutes interval session on a mode of exercise of your choice. Do not do any more than this. Too much cardiovascular training on a resistance training day is counterproductive to muscle repair but an intense interval session will not effect it and will be productive. The most effective time to do this would actually be straight after your resistance workouts on tuesdays, thursdays and saturdays as any glycogen stores would be totally depleted after the resistance workout so only fat will be available as fuel source. However you can also do it as a separate session at lunchtime or other end of the day to your main workout. It may suit your schedule to do this HIIT training first thing on resistance day

mornings as it is short. And you may do your resistance workout then at lunchtime or in the evening.

Cardiovascular days :

Follow the same guidelines as per resistance day above but make sure to leave a few hours between your main workout and this extra workout. It may suit you to do one of the workouts first thing in the morning and your second workout at the other end of the day. It is still best to do a HIIT session or intense circuits like the 4 minute ones in the main programme for this optional additional workout. But if you want to do a more LISS type workout that is fine too. Every bit of exercise is going to be beneficial.

I want to stress something very important. Don't do these extra cardio sessions just to get more quantity in. Remember it is quality not quantity that counts for results. I need you 100% focused on the 6 training sessions on the program and focused on giving me 100% in every single session. If you are giving any less then it will impact results in a big way. The danger with planning on doing extra sessions is that you may start just going through the motions while working out. When you are doing a lot it can start feeling like you are always exercising so the mental stimulation is impacted negatively and this carries over to your effort levels whether that is subconsciously or consciously. Be a good judge of how you are feeling and listen to your body. If your body needs a rest then listen. Keep focused on the quality vs quantity rule and prioritise the 6 MSS exercise programme training sessions weekly. It is crucial that you give 100% to the 6 scheduled training sessions. Don't decrease the quality by doing extra sessions. If you complete extra sessions they should be a positive and a bonus not have a negative impact on the scheduled sessions.

Your MSS Resistance Training Programme

I have designed the whole MSS exercise programme so that it can be done at home with minimal equipment. All you need is a barbell/dumbbell set and a gym ball and a step/chair to stand up on and a small step to sit on. This creates a very inexpensive home gym. If you prefer to exercise in the gym just follow the same programme and use a gym ball or a bench – whichever you prefer. Get a small area of the gym or use a vacant exercise studio and have your barbell and weight plates with you and a reebok step as well as using the bench or a high step of some kind to do step ups on. And then you are all set for a good workout. The whole 6 week resistance programme is based on exercises using your bodyweight and the barbell. If you prefer to replace any of the programme exercises with another free weight or a machine based exercise that is fine once it targets the same muscle group and is a compound exercise. Make sense? If unsure or have questions feel free to contact us on social media or email. You can see full contact details on resources page at back of this book.

Complete your resistance training programme on tuesday, thursday and saturday. This programme involves completing a 10 exercise resistance training circuit using the peripheral heart action strategy by alternating between lower and upper body compound exercises.

Commence with a warm up set of 10 repetitions at 50% of the intended hard set weight for each of the first planned workout exercises for legs, chest and back. So for example this could be squats, press-ups and wide barbell rows. The smaller muscles will also be warmed up when warming up the larger muscles as they are compound exercises so no need to warm these smaller muscles specifically.

Aim to complete 10 repetitions on each exercise reaching the point of muscular failure or even beyond if you have a training partner who can spot you. Please note that although we are aiming for 10 repetitions, there will be times when you might reach failure at 8, 9, 12 or 15 repetitions. Reaching the point of muscular failure is the goal with each set. Use the number of repetitions completed in each exercise of the circuit to plan the weight for the following circuit. You may need to decrease or increase reps or you may need to increase or decrease the weight or sometimes both. 10 repetitions is your guideline reps to aim for.

The time under tension(TUT) I want you to follow is 4,0,2,1 – 4 seconds on the eccentric (lowering/easier/stretching) phase, no pause, 2 second on concentric(pushing or pulling depending on exercise), 1 second pause and repeat. On the eccentric phase count as follows : one one – thousand, two one-thousand, three one-thousand, four one-thousand. By doing this you will count a real 4 seconds. When people count 4 seconds it usually lasts about 2 seconds or less. The eccentric phase is the most important phase of every repetition as it is the phase that creates the most muscle microfibre damage. Our goal in every workout is to create as much muscle fibre damage as possible in every set and every workout. Adhering to the TUT is critical for achieving maximum results. So as you reach the point of muscular failure stay mentally strong to keep the TUT as there will be temptation to speed movement up and even "cheat" on technique to get it done.

Maintaining correct technique and completing full range of movement for each repetition is crucial. Stay focused as you near or reach the point of muscular failure. Never sacrifice technique. If you decide to complete the MSS exercise programme in the gym you will notice that the majority of gym goers have horrendous technique. Do not copy. Read my material and watch my exercise demo videos to learn proper technique. There is a link in the resources section to a playlist on my youtube channel with over 80 exercise demonstration videos. In the resources section you will also have access to illustrations and explanations of these exercises.

If you will be training alone either at home or in the gym then reaching the point of muscular failure will still mean going to the point where you can't physically complete another repetition without sacrificing correct technique and TUT. What I want you to do at this point is to hold an isometric contraction (where you are pushing/pulling but no movement like pushing against a wall) for a 2 second count and then complete the eccentric phase as slowly as you possibly can. This will add extra intensity when exercising alone.

For the 6 weeks I would recommend that you buddy up or hire a personal trainer (worth the investment). If you have a training partner then complete the following on each set : once point of failure has been reached complete two assisted repetitions under control (training partner only giving slightest and required assistance to complete the reps) and then complete two eccentric repetitions. This is painful and mentally challenging to complete especially in a controlled way but keep focused on your why and give it your best shot. This amount of muscular overload will accelerate your results. When I won the Body for Life Competition 2004, this is the strategy I used for each set, with 3 assisted and 3 eccentric reps after I had reached point of muscular failure. Then I would immediately superset (where you complete a set of 2 exercises to failure back to back) with a second exercise for the same muscle group again to failure and again with the 2 added intensity strategies. The pain was immense and mentally I was stretched to the limit. However achieving such outstanding results in a short period of time and becoming Body For Life Challenge Champion meant that my efforts paid off and was more worth the pain. In times of challenge remind yourself of your biggest why and focus on the new body that awaits you.

It is very important to have a stopwatch with you during your workouts as the rest periods are really crucial for effectiveness. If you have a training partner or personal trainer let them keep track. Sticking to the recovery periods is important as recovery periods that are too long or too short will effect the speed of your results. Take a 30-second recovery period between exercises and take a 120-second recovery between circuits. No more and no less. Be strict with the recovery periods I have given. During the recovery periods you can either take a total rest or do active rest which means doing a cardio based exercise like jogging on the spot or boxing or something of low to medium intensity. This is optional but all adds to the overall impact on the body and metabolic impact. By having the short rest periods between sets, applying intensity and reaching muscular failure around the 10 repetition mark your body will experience a larger growth hormone release. This is crucial and plays a major role in building lean muscle while also accelerating fat burning.

The full workout routine requires that you complete 3 rounds of the 10 exercise circuit. Your total workout time should be around 50 minutes once you are strict with the rest periods. If you have a training partner and apply the overload techniques I outlined earlier your workout time will be a few minutes longer. If there are days where you can only complete 1 or 2 circuits that is fine. The programme is designed in such a way that you have the option to complete 15/30/45 minute workouts. This way the program suits different lifestyles and circumstances. Even if you consistently complete the programme there are going to be days where circumstances decide that your option is to either do a quick 15 minute workout or make excuses and do nothing. However what matters most is the intensity you work at. Remember quality beats quantity any day.

As I explained in Chapter 6 muscle confusion is one of 3 key factors in effective training and achieving fast lasting results. Our goal is to experience the fastest results in the next 6 weeks correct? Therefore we need to shock the body frequently with muscle confusion for maximum metabolic and muscular stimulation. For this reason we change the workout routine every single training session. Exercises will repeat (there are a limited number after all) but you will never do the exact same workout routine during the next 6 weeks. Each time an exercise repeats make sure to apply the principle of progressive overload. Your training logbook (see resources section) will become your best friend. Use your training logbook to record what weight and repetitions you completed in your workout as well as how intense it felt out of 10. Ideally you should be aiming for a rating of 10 or at least 9 per set if aiming for muscle failure. Then in your pre workout planning session apply progressive overload as you plan the next workout. Does that make sense? Always plan each session in advance and to include progressions. Remember if you fail to plan you plan to fail.

Does the resistance training programme format now make sense? You have access to detailed illustrations and explanations as well as exercise demo videos of the MSS exercise programme exercises in the resources.

MSS Cardiovascular Training Programme

Your Cardiovascular training will be on monday, wednesday and friday. Each workout involves completing 2 parts with a few minutes rest period between them. You start each cardio day with a HIIT session and then follow it with a 4 minute cardio/abs circuit. Like with the resistance training we incorporate muscle confusion by never doing the exact same workout twice during the 6 weeks. The HIIT session will be different each workout and the exercises in the 4 minute cardio/abs circuit will vary each workout too. The 4 minute circuit exercises will repeat but they will always be in different combinations with different exercises each time. This is similar to the mentality around how the PHA resistance workouts are designed. The exercises chosen are the most effective and are combined in a scientific way for maximum metabolic stimulation. Make sure to apply progressive overload each time you repeat an exercise workout to workout.

Start each workout with an initial 3 minute warm up at a medium pace just jogging on the spot, doing arm rotations and you can do a few repetitions of any of the exercises in that particular day's workout. Then go into your HIIT session for that day following the workout plan outlined in the MSS 6 week programme accessible in the resources section. Once part 1 is completed take a short recovery period of a maximum of 2 minutes and then move onto the second part of the workout which is the 4 minute cardio/abs circuit. Once you start the circuit you keep going without break from one exercise to the next until you have completed one minute on each of the 4 exercises. Then take a 30-second rest between each circuit and complete 7 circuits. Total part 2 workout time is 31 minutes. Added to part 1 this means that cardio days will be about 50 minutes total. But again like I said above in the resistance training section all workouts are designed so that you can do anywhere between 15 to 45 minute workouts. So if under pressure time wise you could just do the HIIT session or do 3 or 4 of the 4 minute circuits. If you only have about 30 minutes you might just do the 7 x 4 minute circuits. Do your best to complete each workout in it's entirety but remember again it's about making the best use of the time you have, apply intensity and focus on quality over quantity. You can find illustrations and explanations and video demos of the exercises in the cardio part of the MSS 6 week exercise programme in the resources section.

It is important that you keep a full training diary. Make sure to download the MSS 6 week exercise programme logbook – check the resources section at the back. Taking time for proper planning and review of your workouts is invaluable. Being disciplined with this is what separates the most successful transformations from everyone else. I'll say it again

If you fail to plan
you plan to fail

Something else I am going to say again is that results will depend on implementing the 3 keys – intensity, progressive overload and muscle confusion. MSS is providing a structured programme to follow incorporating a big focus on muscle confusion. It is your job to implement the other 2 keys as you are the only one who can. Without applying intensity and progressive overload MSS will become just another programme not the fat stripping and lean muscle building programme that it is. MSS is undoubtedly the ultimate mind/body/health programme you will ever find for not just fast but lasting results. We want a dramatic transformation but even more important is that this will be your final body transformation journey. It's time to stop the yo-yo madness and psychological warfare you have been putting yourself through on diets, ineffective programmes and believing in false promises.

NOTE on Flexibility Training :

Flexibility is the most neglected aspect of training and never gets the attention it should. We all need to stretch everyday! Even if you don't exercise you need to stretch as your muscles get tight whether you exercise or not. The majority of lower back pain, neck and shoulder pain and even injuries are as a result of poor flexibility. The modern day lifestyle is to blame as the majority of people are in a seated position most of their waking hours whether at home, commuting or working. When you sit like this for hours your muscles, particularly hamstrings and hips plus neck and shoulders, get tight as you sit hunched over. It is a rarity for someone to sit with correct posture. On the flip side if you are very active you also need to stretch regularly. When you exercise regularly it is very important to put some focused time into flexibility training as your muscles tighten from contracting during exercise. So the next questions are when should you stretch? And how?

Stretching immediately after a cardiovascular workout is the most effective time to stretch. Your muscles are warmed up from the blood circulating during the workout and are more elastic as a result. However do not stretch immediately after resistance training. As mentioned previously resistance training creates microfibre tears in the muscle fibers. If you stretch immediately after your workout this will create further tears which will be counterproductive. Your objective following resistance workouts is to start the repair process. The damage should be done in the workout. Therefore the optimal time to stretch on resistance training days is 3 to 4 hours after the workout when the repairing process is well under way.

So to summarise :

Cardio Workouts : Stretch straight afterwards
Resistance Workouts : Stretch 3 to 4 hours following workout

You can access a detailed flexibility manual with illustrations and explanations of stretches for the main muscles on your body as well as a flexibility routine video in the resources section.

Section 3 : Nutrition

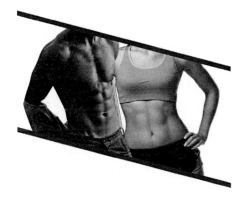

1 – Water : The Surprising Secret To Rapid Fat Loss

Did you realise that your body is made up of 75% water?

Did you realise that water is the MOST important substance that your body needs?

This makes sense when 75% of our bodies are made up of water. Water has an impact on everything that goes on in your body. Another important fact is that our brains are 83% water but crucially our brains do not store water. Therefore when you are not adequately hydrated there will be a big impact on your mood, focus, concentration, memory and all things connected to a healthy brain. What do you think this does to your motivation to exercise and in making the right choices nutritionally? Not being adequately hydrated gives that bad guy in your head even more ammo in the war to turn you into a lethargic, unhealthy, heavily medicated slob with low life quality. You can survive for weeks or even months without food but without water – about a week tops!! Are you now starting to realise just how important water is?

So now that you understand why water is even more important than food I hope this new consciousness will stimulate you to consume more water. The health industry puts so much energy into promoting diets, potions, pills etc with very little mention of water. Most people drink only a fraction of the amount of water they should be drinking but this is largely due to their ignorance to it's many benefits. Now that you have a better understanding that water is important there are many questions that need to be answered like :

1. How much water is enough?
2. Can I drink too much water?
3. Are there recommended times to drink water?
4. What type of water is best?
5. Is tap or bottled water best?
6. Should I invest in one of the many water devices on the market right now?

These are very important questions and I will educate you in detail on the answers throughout this chapter. I will also share my water protocol for safely increasing your daily water intake to the level I recommend.

First I want to educate you on water's impact on your fat levels and explain why I claim it is a secret to rapid fat loss. This is important in keeping with the main focus of this book – transforming your body over the next 6 weeks. There are so many little pieces to the body transformation jigsaw and it will surprise you that water is right up at the top of the list. As I will stress throughout this book, as we put the plan in place for your successful body transformation as well as creating a healthy lifestyle, getting and staying in shape is a lot more than just doing some exercise and dieting. Making positive lifestyle changes and the addition of new habits is the key to lifelong change. So how does water impact fat loss and why did I say it is the secret to rapid fat loss? Let me explain :

Have you ever invested in one of the many, often expensive, detox programmes on the market? There are many and the number available continues to grow as detoxing becomes an industry buzzword and they grow in popularity. I want to tell you that in most cases you are wasting your money unnecessarily. In many cases you worsened your interior environment and only guaranteed short term benefits if experienced some. Why? Because most of these detox concoctions are just creating a more toxic environment when your goal needs to be to make your body less toxic. When you put any chemical compounds or synthetic substances into your body it will make it more toxic. This happens for anything our digestive system is not designed to break down. We are designed to break down wholefood not chemicals. This is why the more removed from wholefood your diet is the more toxic your internal environment is going to be. This applies with medication, processed foods, supplements etc So much of your money ends up being expensive urine and alot remains as toxins and fat deposits (form from collection of toxins) inside your body. Your body creates these fat cells, particularly around the stomach area, to protect the vital organs. Remember your body wants to survive always and will do whatever it feels is best.

The foundational element of an effective and healthy detox plan should be water. Water is free or inexpensive should you take my advice on how to get the highest quality water. More on that later in this chapter. Apart from keeping you hydrated water plays a major role in detoxing your body. When you consume water it hydrates your body and then is excreted via urination while along the way picking up toxins to flush them out your body. The body is truly an amazing and complex specimen. That is why when you take synthetic supplements or medication your urine is usually yellow. Yellow urine may also indicate that you need to drink more water as the darker it is the more dehydrated you typically are. So when your urine is yellow colour analyse your water intake to judge if possibly dehydrated. And if adequately hydrated take a look at your medication and supplement intake in the previous 24 hours. So the upshot of this is that the more water you consume the more you are detoxing your body in a healthy and harmless way.

Apart from my goal to remain hydrated throughout each and every day this is the reason why I consume 6 litres of water daily. That's right 6 litres!! Now before you have a freak attack I want to clarify and stress that I am not expecting you to start consuming 6 litres of water a day right away. This would be very harmful and possibly damaging to your body in particularly your kidneys depending on your current level of water consumption. When you make changes to your water consumption you should make them gradually and get your body used to the new intake and then continue increasing in this way. I am sure, if you are like 99% of people, that you need to consume more water – right? I will be outlining a water consumption protocol shortly but right now I want to make sure you understand that:

1. water is the most important substance you need to put in your body and

2. water should be the foundational element of any detox plan

You may still find it hard to understand why your body may be toxic and why it needs to be flushed daily. You are also likely wondering what all of this has to do with you losing fat and getting in shape. Let me explain this further.

Most people have highly toxic environments in their body. Most people consume diets that include mainly processed and convenient packaged products. These products have tons of ingredients with only a few that are actually wholefood and even the food elements are often heavily processed. The fruits and vegetables you eat, unless organic or self grown, are full of pesticides and chemicals. Sodas are full of chemicals. Junk food is full of chemicals. Stress creates toxins. Alcohol, tobacco and drugs create toxins. Our modern day city environment where we are surrounded by electro magnetic frequencies creates toxins. Laptops, ipads, smart phones, tvs all create toxins from the radiation they put out into our localised environment. Medication creates toxins. Synthetic supplements create toxins.

Exercising is an important way of releasing toxins but also stresses the body and creates free radicals. Then on the flip side you have the many who are totally inactive living the modern lifestyle and without regular exercise there toxic build-up is even worse. So unless you live in the amazon rainforest, living the active life they did hundreds of years ago, you cannot avoid amassing toxins in one or many shapes and forms. I mainly consume a wholefood plant based nutrition plan. I have developed an ability to control my stress levels most of the time. I exercise up to 2 hours or more daily. I am very aware of toxin sources and avoid as much as I can. However even though I am doing a lot right I cannot prevent toxins in my body. Therefore my body is in need of constant detoxification. Now think about yourself and your lifestyle and environment and habits. What in the list above are you exposed to? How toxic do you think your body may be? Now are you starting to realise why using water for detoxification is crucial? Starting to make sense?

You may still be wondering how this relates to fat loss and getting in shape? Quite simple and I briefly referred to it earlier. The level of toxicity in your body impacts how effectively the good stuff you put in is utilised. It also impacts how efficiently the toxins are eliminated from the body. For most people there is an ongoing build-up of toxins due to lifestyle habits and environment as outlined in last paragraph. As these are harmful to the body it stores them as fat cells which typically are on placed on the belly. Hence why belly fat is so common and it is so dangerous. A high level of belly fat is an indicator of a highly toxic body. This is why when you detox properly you notice an immediate decrease in belly fat. So the good news is that much of your belly fat is just a result of toxins and that a focused detox plan (immediate and ongoing) will see an immediate difference in your belly fat levels. You will experience results just by following a water consumption plan even without any changes to your nutritional and exercise habits. Is this starting to make sense now?

So how much water should you drink?

Simple answer is much more than you are consuming right now but let's get more specific. I want you to get to a "lifestyle" where you are consuming 4 litres of water daily. Then when this has become a habit you can take steps to consume closer to 6 litres should you wish. Our starting point is your current water consumption. So for example if you currently consume 1 litre of water daily then for the next 7 days I want you to consume 1 and 1/2 litres of water daily. Once you complete this step then consume 2 litres of water daily for the next 7 days. Our goal is creating a new positive habit so gradual increases work best. Typically from working with clients all over the world I have found that this level of weekly progress is not difficult to follow. Remember your body needs and wants water. It always craves what it needs. Much of the time when you think you are hungry you are actually thirsty. The brain gets the exact same signal whether it is hunger or thirst. Therefore the brain can't differentiate between them and often we think we are hungry when much of the time we are dehydrated. So next time you feel hungry have a glass of water and if 20-30 minutes later you still feel "hungry" you are. Make sense?

Here is my water protocol for getting your water consumption up to 4 litres based on a starting consumption of 1 litre per day :

Current Consumption 1 litre per day

From day 1 to 7 consume 1 and 1/2 litres daily
From day 8 to 14 consume 2 litres water daily
from day 15 to 21 consume 2 and 1/2 litres water daily

from day 22 to 28 consume 3 litres water daily
from day 29 to 35 consume 3 and 1/2 litres water daily
from day 36 to 42 consume 4 litres water daily

Adjust the water protocol guidelines based on what your personal starting point is. What matters most is that you gradually increase your consumption on a weekly basis so your body can adjust. For the rest of your life commit to consuming a minimum of 4 litres of water daily!

Whenever your consumption decreases remind yourself of what you have now learned regarding how big a role water plays in your body. The impact of this increased water consumption will be immediate on your energy, alertness, mood and overall sense of wellbeing as well as on your belly fat levels. This will happen even if you change nothing else in your lifestyle.

I am regularly contacted by people putting the following argument forward :

"too much water is bad for you and your kidneys and can cause serious damage"

My simple response is a resounding NO! But I must stress the importance of following the guidelines and protocol I laid out earlier. If you are consuming 1 litre of water daily for years and then suddenly start consuming 6 litres of water daily it will place a huge extra demand on your body and you will likely experience some or even extreme discomfort. Such a dramatic change in your consumption will place a huge demand on the kidneys. Extremes in anything in life are rarely good even when you are creating positive habits. I prefer to recommend small improvements with the goal of making them lifelong habits. This is why I am so determined to get you out of the diet mentality.

If you follow the protocol outlined increasing your daily water intake eventually to 4-6 litres in the coming weeks and months your body will naturally adjust to the increasing demands. As I said in Section 2 your body has an incredible ability to adapt. This is no different with regard to increasing your water consumption once done smartly with a long term objective. The body is truly amazing in it's ability to adapt to anything – good or bad!! So this is why my answer is always a resounding NO to that argument as once someone uses common sense there will never be problems. How could there be? Water is natural. Water is the most important substance for our bodies. Why would the body not welcome more of it?

It annoys me that people will always worry about getting too much of a good thing but rarely go on about getting too much fat, chocolate, takeaways or alcohol which are 100% guaranteed to cause a negative result. The bottom line is learn to listen to your body. Your body is very smart and it always communicates with you. If you are consuming too much of anything it will let you know. The same applies if you were to dramatically increase your protein intake – you will experience a big increase in your number of excretions daily. Adjust your consumption of water, as with any substance, should it appear that it is placing too much pressure on your system. Then gradually increase consumption where advised and make it a habit. Allow your body time to adjust to accommodate changes. Make sense?

The next question I get asked is

"Are there specific times of the day that you should consume water?"

The answer is yes.

Everybody should be consuming a litre of water first thing each morning. On waking you likely have not had water for between 8 to 12 hours (or longer for those really poor at drinking water). This means that on waking you are in a severely dehydrated state. Therefore your first action each morning should be consuming water. I recommend to start with a glass of water and lemon and then consume the remainder about 5 to 10 mins later. The lemon and water is important to re-alkalise the body after sleep. Apart from it's rehydrating benefit water is energy to the body and brain. You will experience increased energy and alertness in both your body and brain after you consume this litre of water first thing each morning. I can't stress enough how important this action step is each morning. You will experience a difference in your focus, memory, concentration, alertness and overall productivity in completing this simple action step each morning.

I'd advise you to have water with you all day whether a bottle in your car, in your bag or on your desk. You should sip water throughout the day. You can drink water right up to bedtime but be prepared to wake once or twice to go to the toilet. Ideally you don't want to wake up during the night for the toilet as interrupted sleep in a negative as you will find out in Section 4 which is dedicated to sleep. Therefore I would advise drinking water up to within about 2 to 3 hours of bed. This way you should urinate once or twice before bed and then have an uninterrupted sleep.

I find it annoying when people complain that drinking more water will mean taking bathroom breaks all day – so what!! Do you want to experience optimal health, energy and vitality or not? This question shouldn't even need to be asked. Isn't the inconvenience of frequently urinating worth experiencing optimal health via hydration and constant detox? I love the inconvenience of going to the toilet all the time as it means that my body is flushing out toxins all the time. The less toxic my body the healthier and more energetic I will be and so it proves. What do you want?

You should consume water before, during and after all training sessions. When you exercise you are dehydrating through your internal sprinkler system sweat. Therefore it is really important to keep topping up so you remain hydrated. When this becomes habit consuming 1 to 2 litres of water during this pre/during/post workout period becomes routine. Once you do anything for up to 30 days it becomes a lifestyle habit.

There is a time you should **NEVER** drink water. This is during meals and even within 30 minutes either side of the meal. By drinking water during your meal you are losing valuable nutrients as the water completes it's role of continuously flushing the system so many nutrients are going to be grabbed and flushed out. Many valuable nutrient will end up in your urine. What a waste. So stop drinking water 30 minutes before the meal and then resume drinking water 30 minutes after the meal.

You are consuming food to get valuable nutrients into your body. Don't waste them!!

The next question I get asked is

"What type of water is best – tap or bottled?"

This is a difficult question as the real answer is neither. It really is 50/50 between them depending on how you look at each as they both have big negatives. Let me explain why and then I will give you both a FREE solution and a second solution which I recommend you invest in. This will dramatically improve your water quality and your ability to drink water. This investment option will pay back tenfold in the benefits as it has done for my family.

Tap water must come out of the tap at a PH of 7.365 – this is law. However where the water starts at the water plant is nowhere near this PH and is typically highly acidic. Water is recycled so when you see the rivers around your city and see sewerage going in that is where water starts from before being moved to the water plant to get it ready for human consumption. I have visited water plants and the smell is beyond belief. Next in order to meet quality standards our water is filled with chlorine, fluoride and a whole cocktail of chemicals to get it to a stage where it comes out of your tap at 7.365. So when you consume tap water you are also consuming chlorine, chemicals and most worryingly fluoride which has been proven to cause and be a contributor to many diseases and health issues.

Next let's take a look at bottled water which these days is much more preferred by the majority to tap water as a result of growing awareness of what tap water is and also brilliant marketing by bottled water companies. Bottled water is meant to be spring water put in a bottle and this is what the marketing tells you and you are are sold on this. The reality is that most bottled water is just tap water as has been revealed in recent months. Besides this shocker water becomes or already was dead water when bottled. Add to this that most bottled water sits in a warehouse for a period of time (sometimes could be a year!!) after being transported often long distances and then eventually sits on the shelves in supermarkets and shops. In warehouses the water is often exposed to sunlight for periods of time which leads to the plastic from the bottle seeping into the water. So when you drink bottled water you are usually also consuming harmful plastic and also oestrogenic hormones too. Scary stuff.

So back to the dilemma of which should you choose? It's 50/50 if choosing as both are not good. I don't believe either is a clear winner. The dilemma you are left with then is that you need to consume water. So what should you do? Well the fact is clear from this chapter that you must get water into your body and in the quantities I have recommended. You are still better getting water into your body even if it means tap or bottled water being used. When you choose one of these options it becomes even more important that you focus on the quality of your choices with regard to other liquids and the foods you consume. It is crucial that you consume lots of antioxidants, vitamins and minerals which will combat the negative impact of bottled or tap water as they do with all the bad guys attacking your body. It is the same as how these food counteract bad foods being consumed. Of course the more good things you do the better but at least if you are counteracting some negative habits with positive ones you are doing something to counteract. Remember your body is like a battleground and you want antioxidants, vitamins and minerals to defeat the free radicals and toxins in your body. You need to outnumber them to win the war.

I mentioned earlier that I would give you a both a FREE solution and one that requires an investment to solve your water dilemma. So here they are.

FREE :

Fill glass jugs with tap water and leave them sit for up to 24 hours before consuming. When in the open air chlorine and some chemicals in the tap water will start to disperse so after 24 hours you are then left with fairly clean pure water apart from the fluoride and chloramine which you need certain devices attached to your tap to eliminate. So this is an ok solution and better than drinking straight from the tap or bottled water. It's free. However the water will lose it's charge, life and energy but at least will be decent fairly clean water. It will be much better than tap or bottled water. So go with this option versus straight from tap or bottled water.

Investment :

In 2010 I had been researching water for a couple of years having identified and realised just how important it was for our overall health, performance, results, optimised brain function and basically everything that goes on in our body and even brain as I have shared. The more I learned the more fascinated I became and was truly shocked with what I learned about tap water and especially bottled water. The bottled water industry illustrates the power of marketing and also I have to acknowledge the genius of whoever started bottled water. From my research I grew to understand that our water needs to be charged. I also learned that consuming alkaline ionised water is the optimum water to consume. The word alkaline is key here. As I have stressed throughout this nutrition section we need to consume predominantly alkaline based food and liquids. Remember the more alkaline your consumption is the more efficiently your body will operate and the greater protection you have from all diseases. The fact is that disease cannot survive in an alkaline environment. This is powerful. Add to this the impact of alkaline ionised water on our fat levels which i came to realise. This is when I started to explore the options around the globe for alkaline ionised water and while there are many options (as with any solution in product/device form) there was only one that ticked all the boxes – the Kangen Alkaline Water Ionizer.

Our investment in a Kangen Alkaline Water Ionizer is one I look upon as possibly the best investment I have ever made but is definitely the #1 investment I have made in both my own and my family's health. Once you experience Kangen water you fully understand from the first mouthful just how bad tap and bottled water actually are. While tap and bottled water feels like it is sloshing around your belly Kangen water just flows through and is easy to drink with no water belly. The molecular structure is completely different which allows for quick absorption into the body. I am not going to get into this in depth as I could write a whole book on water and my research and what I have learned as well as my experience using Kangen Alkaline Ionised water. My goal here is to make you aware of it and if you would like to learn more about it check out the resources section at the back of the book for links to websites, videos and also some documents explaining it's many benefits and direct comparisons to other ionisers as well as methods/devices for improving water quality.

In my opinion every household in the world needs a kangen alkaline water ioniser installed. I have set up a dedicated website:

www.kangenwateristhebestalkalinewater.com   where you can see loads of information about it. Should you have any questions our would be interested in investing in a unit contact me by email or via one of our social medias and we can arrange to discuss.

Summary :

We have covered a lot in this chapter and I expect that you are surprised by how much there is to know about water. Like I stated at the start of this chapter most are totally unaware of just how important water is. Keep remembering that our bodies are composed of 75% water and our brains 83%. We must remain hydrated and even 1 week without water is fatal. Your goal is in the coming weeks to get your consumption to 4 litres a day following my water protocol. Go do it. It is your most important first step in this journey.

2 – Intermittent Fasting :
A Fad Or Worth Doing?

My first exposure to the concept of intermittent fasting was about 4 years ago when a client emailed asking my thoughts on this new concept they had seen recommended on some website. What got them curious was that a friend of theirs was following it with impressive results. My initial reaction was dismissive. My reaction still is to a degree. Now there a wide array of versions of intermittent fasting being recommended by "experts". I.F. has grown like many new concepts, devices or gimmicks that launch in the weightloss and fitness world.

When the concept was first brought to market it became fashionable and popular. Then many "experts" jumped on the bandwagon and just tweaked the initial core concept a little, putting their own unique but unscientific spin on it. So firstly I am going to tell you to beware of I.F. and all the versions that are out there. When my client contacted me I took a look at I.F. in more details so that I could give them a proper point of view on it. Some of the plans were very extreme. Someone I knew was following a particular I.F. plan which meant having 3 days consuming about 400 calories and then a day consuming as much as you want of any type of food. It is 100% wrong to consume so few calories and I don't care if it was only 3 days before a binge. The human body has no reason to be put under such dramatic strain and stress unless in a famine or another holocaust situation. Such a plan is just not right and is not good for your body. At the time the majority of plans were extreme like this which meant I then ignored I.F. and advised my client not to dare touch it. I labelled it as yet another stupid dangerous fad.

In recent years I.F. has again grown in popularity and has been getting a lot of media coverage. Naturally, as someone who keeps their finger on the pulse of the industry, my attention was drawn to a few new I.F. plans as well as developing a desire to research it deeper. I have always been a fairly open minded individual and have never just believed in people's opinions without researching myself and as a result forming my own opinion. I would never and have never in over 20 years recommended anything to clients unless I have personally been a guinea pig myself for it and had positive results from it. Also of great importance on top of results is that what I would have researched on it must have made sound scientific and real life sense. Then it gets my seal of approval.

Now based on the knowledge I have acquired from researching for the last couple of years I now definitely see a place for I.F. but only certain plans and only for certain people. The main reason for it's popularity and it's marketing strategy is all centered around the rapid body fat loss it is claimed to cause. Anything that claims to lose fat fast gets attention. This is why so many I.F. programmes have made their creators a fortune. The majority will experience short term success and popularity as they are too difficult to follow. Let's leave the possible body fat benefit aside for a moment as what is most important is understanding what impact I.F. has on your body and its functions. Are there any concrete reasons to follow such a plan?

In today's world we consume a lot of processed and convenient food. The world has done so for a long time now. Humans have moved from growing their own fruits and vegetables and making family dinners from scratch to relying on ready made meals, boxed pizzas and microwaves. This is the current reality in a large percentage of households on the planet. Then add to that the amount of chemicals and pesticides that are now sprayed on or added to our food in it's growth and production. Unless you grow your own food or eat only organic the digestion system is fighting a lot of new battles every time you consume food and liquids. This change in our lifestyle means that our digestive systems are under dramatically increased pressure compared to our relatives decades or centuries ago. Also our drinking water is now so much more toxic as shared in the previous chapter. Stress and environmental factors are further sources of toxins for the body to deal with.

Now as a result of what I shared in the previous paragraph I see a role for I.F. both for health and accelerating fat loss. When our digestive systems are under so much pressure it is impossible for it to process everything efficiently and our bodies are constantly being filled with toxins. Colons get blocked. Kidneys get overworked. Stomachs and the whole digestive and excretory systems are under too much pressure. Regular bowel movements are no longer common with most people. You should be going for #2 at minimum twice a day and even better 3 or 4 times daily. You also should be urinating frequently once your water intake is adequate. Toxins need to come out and the digestive and excretory systems need to work as they are designed to in order to meet this need. If we focus on body fat a build-up of toxins leads to a build-up of fat cells as toxins are combined together and fat cells created especially on the stomach. So the end result is that you can be exercising like your life depends on it and consuming a fantastic plant based wholefood diet but modern life means that it is now more difficult to burn fat and shift stored fat – make sense?

There are just 2 I.F. plans that I am ok with people following. They both give your digestive system a break allowing you body time to flush out the toxins and you will also experience a decrease in body fat especially around the stomach area.

24 Hour Intermittent Fasting :

This one is tough but is very rewarding for your digestive and excretory systems as well as from body fat decrease point of view. When I did my #30daysbacktosixpack for the month of November in 2015 I included this strategy into my plan to test it out. I did 5 days following a nutrition programme and then a 24 hour I.F. I usually started the fast around lunchtime and finished lunchtime the next day. It sure was tough especially the first time but while it never got easy it got more bearable. You can pick any 24 hour period with the most popular typically from around 7pm at night to the following evening at 7pm and then a big feed. This way one is usually going to bed soon after starting so a large chunk of hours used up during that period until get up the following morning. I did notice a difference in body fat levels from implementing this in my plan. However it is not something I would do regularly as just didn't suit me and how it made me feel. But it is effective if you are happy to follow it. Some incorporate one 24 hour fast into each week. Personally I feel it is an effective strategy to implement maybe once every few months to give your digestive system a break.

8 Hour Eating Window & 16 Hour Fast:

This I.F. plan has become quite popular and I am not surprised it has. I know of many who follow it religiously and love it and have experienced great results. It is a plan you follow every day vs sporadically. It does go against some of my fat loss strategies with such a long fasting time daily and eating as much as you want during those 8 hours. However it does make some sense in terms of giving digestive system time to break down our food. I am not for or against this plan but if it felt right for you then go for it and give it a go. Usually you would fast starting between 4-6pm and then until 10am the next morning. Then between 10am and 4-6pm you would eat whatever you want and as much as you want. I think this has become appealing especially to those who have got into the bad habit of not eating a breakfast for many years and also those who love eating massive quantities of food when they do it.

In summary I wanted to include a chapter on I.F. to share my thoughts on this type of plan as it has become popular. Personally I would not follow either apart from a 24 hour fast a few times a year to give my digestive system a total break. But I am not against anyone following either plan. They are the only 2 I.F. plans that I can see some logic and benefits in following. Make up your own mind about what suits you. Should you decide you want to follow one of them get in touch with us so we can advise how to tweak your MSS nutrition plan as like I said I.F. goes against many of the principles and strategies our foundation is build on.

3 – Take Positive Steps :My Top 15 Nutritional Dos

In this chapter I will outline my top 15 Nutritional Dos. Notice how they are "dos" not "don´ts"!! This is important so pay attention to what I am going to say next. When making changes in your lifestyle it is important that you focus on adding and taking positive steps versus being told "don't" do this and that. Don't creates negative energy which implies deprivation. Whether you are a child or an adult you don't react well to being told not to do something. This usually leads to you wanting to do it like the way people seem to always want what they can't have. Make sense? Can you relate? We want to create positive energy around your whole journey. This is very important in relation to your attitude towards food as so much of our lives revolve around food. Popular diets are all focused on eliminating and lead to deprivation whereas the right approach is to focus on adding not taking away. Does this sound like a better approach? You are going to find out during the next 6 weeks.

Do #1 : Eat a breakfast every morning :

Breakfast is the most crucial meal of the day because as the word itself reveals you "break" the "fast". When you wake up, depending on your eating and sleeping habits, you will have gone anything up to 12 hours without any food. Therefore you need to fuel up for the day ahead. You wouldn't expect to be able to drive a car without petrol or diesel would you? So you need to get energy into your body from the start and then your job is to maintain this energy supply throughout the day but more on that in Do #2. In terms of our goal of fat loss stimulating your metabolism is always your goal and when you eat you stimulate your metabolism by kicking your digestive system into gear and the digestive process burns a lot of calories – make sense? So eating stimulates your metabolism. It is no different to putting fuel into a fire. After you eat the body breaks your food down and then supplies energy for your body and brain to function throughout the day. So think of breakfast as lighting up a fire. Breakfast typically should be your second action step each morning at least 15 minutes after rehydrating with a litre of water. However there is one exception to this rule. If you decide to exercise first thing in the morning in a fasted state, as I recommend, then eat your breakfast 30 to 60 minutes post workout. Immediately post workout is when your body burns the most calories, once stimulated correctly, so don't waste this opportunity by eating straight away. Remember your goal is to burn as much fat as possible not to refuel immediately after workouts as would be the protocol for endurance or strength athletes.

Do #2: Eat at least 4 to 5 times a day :

This should be great news for you. If you are a serial dieter then you are used to being told to eat very little or in a very restricted way eliminating loads of foods. On the MSS nutrition programme you get to eat a lot of food but in a structured way. Many people still follow the typical three square meals a day and so many people follow popular diets rife with deprivation and calorie counting. They also have a negative impact on your psychology. Such plans have a negative impact on your metabolism so are not good long term strategies. Remember our focus is on keeping your metabolism as elevated as possible each day and elevating your basal metabolic rate. This is a key part of our strategy to experience lifelong results not short term. Having massive gaps between meals becomes a bad habit with "busy" people. Some even have 8 hour gaps between their lunch and their dinner. Working through lunch or taking care of kids or getting distracted often takes priority over fuelling your body. This needs to stop. In Do #1 above I compared having breakfast to lighting up a fire. Now think about this. Once the fire is blazing do you just leave it until it is dead again and light it up again? Or do you top it up every time the flames go down and reach a point where less heat being given off? Your body is no different when we speak of stimulating your metabolism and creating energy. Also don't forget your brain consumes 20% of the calories you consume and needs to be constantly fuelled. It is the most active muscle in your body despite taking up only 2% of your bodyweight. Your brain burns fuel fast and therefore needs regular feeding. Frequent eating therefore burns more calories, keeps energy levels high and ensures optimal brain function. There is only one exception and that is if you decided to follow one of the two Intermittent Fasting methods discussed in the previous chapter. If you decide to do this make sure to eat frequently during your eating window. To clarify I am not recommending I.F. but it is a strategy I would have no problem in you following once you do it right as I instructed in that chapter.

Do #3. Eat 5 portions of fruit, vegetables and salad per day.

There is way too much focus on how much protein we need to consume especially when we don't need a fraction of what the food and supplement industry tell us we do. We will go into more detail about our macronutrient requirements later in this section. Your fruits and vegetables intake is far more important to focus on as they are your source of vitamins, minerals and antioxidants. These food sources need to be the foundation of your daily nutrition programme if you are to achieve maximum results and improve your health at the same time. Pay particular attention to your daily consumption of green vegetables like kale, spinach, cucumber, broccoli, wheatgrass etc. These are full of chlorophyll which rather than protein is the most beneficial for recovery. Aim to consume at minimum 5 portions of fruits and vegetables daily. You can easily achieve this in smoothies and a wide variety of meals. You will have access to recipes for snacks and meals in the resources section of this book.

Do #4. Eat good fats daily.

All fats are not equal and some are beneficial even for increased fat loss. There are both good fats and bad fats. Avoid the bad fats which are saturated and trans fats which are included in most processed food and confectionary. Saturated fats are very high in animal protein particularly red meat. During the next 6 weeks you will be following a plant based nutrition plan so you will benefit a lot with a decreased saturated fat intake. I recommend that you eat good fats daily i.e omega 3,6 and 9. Sources include avocados, nuts, nut butters, seeds and oils (preferably olive oil and coconut oil). Please note that fats contain 9 calories per gram so be mindful of this in your consumption of them particularly with oils. There is no problem consuming good fats but you must beware of overdoing it.

Do #5. Learn to read food labels and learn the truth about low fat and low sugar foods

During the last few decades there have been phases of low fat marketing. In recent times there has been a shift towards demonising sugar. Each phase has seen the introduction of free from and no fat/sugar product ranges. The food industry is clever and moves with the trends and with what will make the most profit. Remember my message in #4 that bad fats are not good but all fat are not equal so just because something has fat in it does not mean it is bad. The same with sugar as there are various forms of sugar good and bad. If it is highly refined then it is not good for us but if it is coming from fruit then it is. The quality and benefit of food products depends on the level of processing it has gone through. The more impact man has had in creating the final product the worse it becomes!! Don't be fooled by marketing. While the front of a product may give a positive healthy message – like low fat, low sugar, no fat/sugar – it is the back of the product that tells the full story. Much of the time, while it may not have fat and/or sugar, it will instead have loads of artificial sweeteners, E numbers and chemicals added so it still tastes good and for shelf life. Remember if the product does not taste good it will not sell. So if you take out the fat and/or sugar the product will taste terrible if nothing is added. Therefore they add lots of different forms of sugar as well as chemicals to low/no fat products and add artificial sweeteners and E numbers to low/no sugar products. The closer a food is to it's original or natural form the better it will be. If you are going to buy any packaged food make sure to learn how to read nutritional labels on the back of products.

Do #6. Eat nutritionally balanced meals

Our bodies need a wide variety of both the macro and micronutrients each day. Vitamins, minerals, carbohydrates, protein, fats and fibre all have important roles to play in our body. Therefore each time you eat aim to have as many of the different nutrients included as possible. Always consume a portion of carbohydrates at every meal as like I have previously stated it is our body and brain's source of energy. That is it's only function and it's an important one. However be careful with the quantity and type of carbohydrate you consume. Balance is important with your meals. Carbohydrate sources contain varying degrees of sugar which has the effect of elevating blood sugar and insulin levels. When a high sugar carbohydrate source is chosen your insulin level will elevate substantially, then drop dramatically and then your body craves more high sugar carbohydrates in order to return to neutral. However this usually results in a vicious circle if high sugar carbohydrates are continuously chosen. Not only will this effect your energy levels but it will also lead to increased risk of fat storage. This is why it is important to have protein and foods rich in fibre containing fruit, vegetables and salad with your meals. These foods slow the release of the sugars from the carbohydrates. In each meal have a portion of carbohydrates and protein and in as many meals as possible have vegetables and salad. Consume fat with 1 or 2 meals and typically eat fruit on it's own or 30 minutes before a meal as it digests the fastest so needs to be eaten first or it will just sit on the other food and rot in the stomach.

Do #7. Consume a minimum of two litres of water daily.

As you learned in chapter one of this section our bodies are made up of 75% water. That chapter stressed a lot of reasons why water is crucial to both your body and brain. Consuming a minimum of 2 litres of water a day is a critical part of your nutritional plan. This should be an absolute minimum as like I recommended in chapter one you should aim to get your daily consumption to 4 litres a day. Follow the water protocol I outlined in Chapter one of this section to increase your water intake and make it a positive habit. As you learned water plays an important role in all of the functions and systems of the body. Make sure you remain hydrated throughout each day. Water detoxifies the body flushing out the waste products and toxins. High intakes of water each day will increase your fat burning ability especially around the midsection where a lot of toxins are stored as belly fat.

Do #8. Eat wholefood plant based foods :

As I will explain in chapter 8 eating wholefood plant based food is the best choice for many reasons including increased fat loss (particularly around the belly area), gaining lean muscle, improved energy, improved brain function, improved performance and recovery and much more. The benefits are many but for the purposes of this book's focus fat loss and metabolic stimulation are key ones. In the next 6 weeks you are going to experience much fat loss just from following a wholefood plant based nutrition plan. Chapter 7 will clarify a lot for you as I will be sharing much of what I have learned about a plant based lifestyle.

Do #9. Allow your body time to digest for the last 4 hours before sleep and prevent possible fat gain.

If you want to increase your body fat percentage fast, eating before bed, is the most effective strategy you can use. Make sure you read that line again so you don't misunderstand it! All food sources take different times to digest and get broken down. Typically most plant based foods will take up to 3 hours to digest. Red meat can take days!! This is why in Do #2 I recommended eating 4 or 5 times a day which means about every 3 hours. In the evening you are less active and usually relaxing and winding down mentally and physically. For this reason you don't have the same energy requirements as during the day. So it is advisable to leave 4 hours between your final meal and sleep. At the end of the day your body does a stocktake and any excess carbohydrate are temporarily stored in your liver. These will then convert to fat within a few days if your lifestyle does not require calling on reserves. This is the case for most unless an elite endurance athlete exercising 3 hours a day. So I recommend you don't eat within four hours of bed. Allow your body time to digest and break down the food consumed during the day. Also eating before bed impacts your sleep quality and as you will read in Section 4 quality sleep is key to results.

Do #10. Enjoy your favourite treat/reward/luxury foods once a week

In all of my products and coaching I always recommend the use of a reward meal each week. Notice again the positive language. Instead of "cheat" meal I said "reward" meal. I want you to see it as a reward for sticking to your plan during the week. It is important that you incorporate a mental and physical break from a strict nutrition plan. For your reward meal decide on something you really enjoy having – could be a pizza, takeaway, ice cream, cake or could be going for a few drinks. Personally I love having a chocolate cake or cookies with ice cream.

NOTE – it does not have to be food. Reward could be clothes or a massage. I usually refer to food as typically most people's lives revolve around food.

Do #11. Replace processed foods which are full of sugar, salt and preservatives.

The modern lifestyle is all about convenience. Unfortunately this has resulted in people eating more and more processed foods. Fresh wholefood has been replaced by boxes and cans. Once a product is inside a can, bottle, container or a box it typically contains preservatives, high quantities of refined sugar, salt and chemicals and additives to prolong shelf life. Basically the more man has played a part in the final product the more processed it will be. Sometimes products contain ingredients which we have never heard of and can't even pronounce. Decreasing or ideally eliminating processed foods will make a huge difference to your waistline and health. Remember anything your body can't break down will usually become toxic in the body and will then lead to fat cells being created and becoming belly fat. These foods are a major reason for both fat gain and also your body holding onto fat instead of burning it as your body's efficiency slows down. Keep your food as clean and fresh as you can. Try to eat fresh, ideally organic food where possible. Focus on consuming a nutrition plan largely made up of fruits, vegetables, salads, berries, nuts, seeds, legumes, grains etc. I would advise you to use this program to avoid all processed food, create this positive habit and likely continue it beyond finishing this programme. You want to flush out toxins and any water retention not add to it.

Do #12. Enjoy social occasions without alcohol.

I can hear you screaming NO!! I am going to start by reminding you that we are only talking about a 6 week commitment for the duration of this programme. You can decide then what you would like to do at the end of it. Be willing to do whatever it takes to achieve results and making sacrifices is always key to success in any area of life. Don't drink alcohol for the next 6 weeks. Alcohol is the # 1 sabotager of results especially when your target is stripping fat from around the mid-section.

Alcohol is not a nutritional source so therefore contains empty calories which are converted to sugar and then typically fat cells. Alcohol increases your blood sugar level resulting in food cravings. This is why we have the urge to eat during and after alcohol. The next day hangovers continue your craving for unhealthy fatty and sugary food. The overall effect of alcohol is detrimental to results. Remember your nutrition plays the greatest role in your body transformation so alcohol converting to fat cells and also increasing your "bad" food consumption is not going to help. The quality of your sleep is also negatively effected as you are unable to reach the rapid eye movement phase of sleep which is critical to rest and recuperation. If your sleep quality is effected so too are your results. And as you will learn in Section 4 continued poor sleep results in cortisol release and this further increases fat cells especially around the stomach. Making this sacrifice with alcohol for the next 6 weeks will be more than worth the benefits and results.

Do # 13. Replace tea and coffee

This is another one that you may not be happy with. However tea and coffee serve no purpose nutritionally and only cause negative effects with the caffeine. You can also grow a huge dependence on coffee which is evident all over the world with addiction clearly evident in many cases. I want you to cleanse your body and to truly fuel it with energy via foods that provide "real" energy. So instead of having coffee or tea drink water ideally but if you want a hot drink then have green tea (loaded with antioxidants and also is a thermogenic so increases metabolism and fat burning) or peppermint tea which is great for digestion or late at night camomile tea is great to relax. Coffee also stresses the adrenal glands which is another reason for fat gain. Coffee stimulates the adrenal glands, which means that every time you drink coffee, you're activating the body's fight-or-flight response. But, instead of releasing adrenaline so the body can react to a true stressor, the adrenals are releasing this hormone in response to your coffee consumption.

Do # 14. Keep insulin levels more stable by replacing soft drinks and flavoured water

Soft drinks are a disaster when it comes to losing fat and getting in shape. They are loaded with sugar. A can of coke contains 12 spoons of sugar!! That's right 12 – hard to comprehend and this fact tends to shock people. So in our process of cleansing and detoxing your body it is important to eliminate soft drinks. During the next 6 weeks any soft drinks consumed will impact results and due to high sugar content will increase your chance of actually gaining fat on your body due to the impact on your insulin levels as well as excess calories being stored!! Flavoured waters are not good either and just popular due to clever marketing. I must also mention energy drinks like red bull and monster and their equivalents are disastrous too. Anything that is loaded with refined sugars of various types, chemicals and ingredients you have no idea what they are should be avoided and eliminated. So avoid all and drink water instead or a smoothie!!

Do #15. If you do want to use supplements then use wholefood plant based ones

I speak in detail about supplements and the industry in Chapter 8 of this section. I used to use synthetic supplements for about 20 years but haven't used any since about 2010 once I learned the truth about the industry and about the quality of ingredients being used in the products. Synthetic means man made and majority of supplements are chemical compounds combined to create a substance that is designed to replicate a food source or vitamin or mineral. These are not the actual nutrients – just replicas. Our bodies are designed to break down real wholefood and not such ingredients. Our digestive system has a hard time digesting anything synthetic and a lot of the time these products end up being just expensive urine or remain in the body making it more toxic. I have seen many x-rays which revealed a number of capsules in someone's stomach as the body was unable to break them down!! If you are going to add any supplements to your nutrition plan make sure they are wholefood and plant based as well. You will learn loads more about this whole topic in Chapter 8.

4 – *Light The Fire Within You*

Our goal with the MSS programme is to elevate your metabolism as high as possible as this will lead to greater calorie burning. When I mention metabolism in previous sentence I am referring to both your metabolic rate throughout the day and your basal metabolic rate. What are both of these?

Your basal metabolic rate is :

The rate at which the body uses energy while at rest to maintain vital functions such as breathing and keeping warm.

Whereas when I refer to your metabolic rate during the day I mean :

The rate at which you are burning calories at various times during that day.

This will be impacted by both your nutrition and exercise habits during that day. In section 2 I explained in detail how exercise elevates your metabolism during the day as well as elevating your basal metabolic rate as you get fitter and increase your lean muscle mass. Your nutritional can also impact your metabolic rate throughout the day. As well as consuming food for fuel our goal with food is also increasing metabolism as both our digestive and energy systems are kicked into gear. When you follow effective nutritional strategies, such as you will learn in this section, it will result in an increase in calories burned throughout each day, week and month. Achieving a faster basal metabolic rate and keeping your metabolism elevated throughout each day will see you stripping fat fast, building lean muscle and easily maintaining your new body shape once it is achieved. In the last section I explained how exercise plays a critical role in creating a faster metabolism. Now let's get into the specifics of why and how your nutritional habits can also create a faster metabolism so you can maximise your daily calorie burning potential.

In the previous chapter I outlined 15 nutritional Dos and 2 of them included always eating breakfast and eating every 3 hours. In our fast paced world so many people regularly skip breakfast and tend to consume food sporadically with no structure to their daily eating habits. Not only is this disastrous for their energy and brain function but also has a huge impact on their fat levels and overall body shape and health. Not having breakfast and consuming infrequent meals with long gaps between meals leads to lowering your metabolic rate throughout the day and this in turn contributes to slow or minimal fat loss while following an exercise programme. Remember your nutrition plays an 80% role in any body transformation plan.

Let me explain the importance of breakfast again. By breakfast I mean your first meal of the day. I specify that as this could mean you eating 15 minutes after you get up or a couple hours after should you exercise first thing in the morning in a fasted state as I have recommended. If following my maximum results guidelines for the MSS programme breakfast will be 30 to 60 minutes post workout so this could be 2 to 2 and ½ hours after you wake up. In this scenario the workout is the metabolic kicker first thing in the morning versus the breakfast. Remember the comparison I make between your metabolic rate each day and a fire. So at one of the two times you are "break" ing the "fast". That is why it is referred to as breakfast and it is so crucial that you have breakfast as one of first action steps each day. Coffee has become many people's breakfast and is a very poor substitute. So that's breakfast – does that now make sense as to why you need to have one each morning? Your breakfast is like when you light up a fire at the start and have it blazing. Should you exercise first thing that is the start of the fire and then the breakfast raises it up another level. So like a double elevation. This is highly effective routine as your metabolic rate starts off early at a very elevated level. Once you then follow my advice for the rest of the day you will keep it at a high to medium level throughout. This will maximise your calories burned that day.

Each time you eat your metabolic rate elevates like when you add more fuel into a fire when flames are lowering. As I said in the last paragraph once you exercise in a fasted state first, you will experience a double metabolic raise with your breakfast following the initial metabolic impact of your workout. While asleep, your metabolism is much lower as your body is at rest but it still continues to burn calories especially as it is the repairing phase of your day. Throughout each day your basal metabolic rate will continue to tick away. Like I defined earlier your basal metabolic rate leads to energy expenditure energy as needed to meet demands of everything going on in your body and brain. Without a kickstart your metabolic rate would stay low throughout the day thus slowing your progress dramatically due to lower calories being burned.

Now let me explain the need for regular feedings throughout the day. Let's go back to the fire comparison. Once the flames decrease you add more fuel which gets burned up and energy is then given off by way of heat. This process continues, until you let the fire die out late at night. Your body requires the same fuelling process. You add fuel to the fire (food to your body) which is burned up(food broken down and digested) and it gives off heat (your body supplies energy). Your workout and breakfast will kickstart your metabolism first thing each morning as explained earlier. Then in order to maintain high levels of energy and an elevated metabolic rate you need to eat frequently to activate the process outlined above. You achieve this by consuming small balanced meals frequently throughout the day. I recommend every 3 hours or 2 to 2 and ½ if was more a snack or lighter meal. This will then allow the body to burn fuel (calories) and give off energy and maximise the process. For example if you eat your first meal at 7am then your next meal should be at 10am, then 1pm, then 4pm and finally at 7pm. Once you have finished your last meal, which should be close to 4 hours before bed(this example 11pm), your metabolism will gradually slow down until you go to sleep. Can you now understand why I compare keeping your metabolism elevated to the process of lighting and maintaining a fire?

There is a huge difference in the metabolic effect of having breakfast following exercise first thing in the morning plus consuming regular balanced meals every 3 hours versus skipping both exercise and breakfast, having a quick bite at 10am, lunch at 1pm and dinner at 7/8pm which is typical of what many do. Also this second scenario is assuming the individuals are making healthy choices which is often not the case. Bad food will have a negative not a positive impact on your metabolism. Another negative is that when someone eats infrequently they tend to eat very large quantities when they do eat and eat much faster which further slows your metabolism as the body has to focus so much on breaking down and digesting this large quantity of food. Once you have benefited from the early morning kickstart small frequent balanced meals play a vital role in maintaining an elevated metabolism and thus burning a higher level of calories daily.

While frequent meals are important so too is ensuring that they are nutritionally balanced meals. Always have a portion of carbohydrates and protein with each meal and have vegetables and/or salad with as many of the meals as possible. A portion would be as follows :

Imagine a plate for a minute. This is how it should look

- ¼ of the plate should contain carbohydrate
- ¼ protein
- and ½ vegetables and salad.

Would you agree that this is a little different to how people normally portion control their meals? Most people eat a huge portions of carbohydrates with each meal, especially if spaghetti or other pasta or potatoes if Irish. Others eat tons of animal protein in the form of meat. Many claim to not like vegetables and salad or a very limited range of it. Such poor eating habits and portion control is what leads to sluggishness and increasing fat levels. I will be speaking in more detail about these individual nutrients in the next few chapters.

To summarise this chapter the key message is that order to burn as many calories as possible each day never skip breakfast and eat frequent nutritionally balanced meals. Keep thinking of the comparison with how a fire works. I hope that comparison has given you a better understanding of having control over your nutritional programme in coordination with your exercise programme in terms of it's overall metabolic effect.

Higher metabolism = more calories burned = results ONCE you are following a healthy balanced nutrition plan as this section will outline.

5 – *Are Carbs Friend Or Foe?*

There is so much confusion about carbohydrates that I have included a dedicated chapter to clarify things. I am going to share my personal opinion formed from both research and experience. In the last two decades low and no carb diets have become very popular and fashionable. This trend started with the Atkins Diet and the most recent one is Paleo. Some low/no carb diets have been partly healthy in the foods you are allowed eat and had some logic in their arguments but others like the Atkins Diet have been ludicrous, defying logic and so unhealthy in the foods recommended. The Atkins Diet recommended eating mainly foods containing bad fats to make you feel satisfied and to suppress appetite and this then also satisfied one's desire to eat crap food. There is nothing beneficial about eating cheese burgers, fried eggs, processed meats etc. More recently The Paleo Diet has become very popular with a big following with a variety of versions including a plant based vegan paleo diet. The main basis of these diets and what they preach is that carbohydrates are bad and are the reason for fat gain and rising obesity. They also put a huge focus on sugar but what they are not accounting for is like fats there are 2 kinds of sugar – good and bad.

The logic of the Paleo Diet, and all low/no carb diets, is that in eliminating carbohydrates or limiting them substantially you will lose weight rapidly. These are typically ketogenic diets which is where ketones are produced for energy when carbohydrates are really low. Low carb dieting has also been popular for decades in the bodybuilding world in the lead up to a show sometimes with dieting lasting 12 weeks. So is there logic to these diets? Should such a carb cutting strategy be used by mainstream instead of just bodybuilders? Are carbohydrates really that bad? NO to each of the three questions. Carbohydrates are not bad and I capitalised "no" to stress the point. In fact they are a necessary nutrient for the body.

Our bodies are designed to run on carbohydrates or more accurately glycogen which is what carbohydrates are eventually broken down into. Carbohydrates to our body is like petrol/diesel to a car or motorbike. We need them and we need plenty of them. Carbohydrates enable you to function throughout the day, maintain high energy levels and, depending on your goals, complete exercise sessions. They are also crucial to brain function as your brain consumes 20% of the calories you consume with it's preferred energy source being carbohydrates. A plentiful supply allows for better mood, concentration, focus and memory.

Some will claim that fat is our preferred fuel source. This is not totally true but it is true that fat can be used as fuel. Many times it is and since the beginning of time there have been periods where using fat as fuel has ensured survival. However in general we don't want it to be our fuel source. It is very slow releasing and when it is being used as our fuel it makes us feel like crap. If the body stops releasing fat as fuel, should it feel under threat of starvation, it will then move to using protein as energy source which means breaking down muscle. When this happens it shows that the body is in trouble as we never want to lose muscle mass. This is exactly what happens on most diets. The body begins to eat itself via muscle and also withdraws valuable minerals from your bones. Should this continue for a period of time it will lead to both muscle and bone problems and diseases. This is why most of the weight lost on popular diets is actually muscle and bone. Fat will not be used as fuel if the body feels threat of starvation. Your body wants to survive.

On many popular diets people drop incredible weight fast but usually only a small proportion of this weight loss is actually fat. The rest is made up of muscle, bone and water. Dieters are usually left with a slower metabolism and decreased muscle mass and bone density. Not very positive results. Added to that the weight lost is usually gained back twice over within a few months or even weeks. These diets also have a terrible impact on one's mood, memory, concentration, focus and motivation which is a consequence of starving the brain of the carbohydrates it needs for energy to function optimally.

So in general we want to utilise carbohydrates as our fuel source throughout each day but we structure our meal/training timings so that we are using fat as our fuel during workouts. We structure our daily nutrition so we consume enough carbohydrate to feel energetic and alert all day but not so much that we have a calorie surplus at the end of the day. Our goal is a calorie deficit. Is this making sense?

While carbohydrates are important for energy be mindful that excess consumption may lead to fat storage. Your body stores glycogen in the muscles but when these are full excess glycogen is stored temporarily in the liver which if not used within a few days is converted to fat cells. This is why for most the latter will happen as they are not active enough to need to draw on reserves. Another important tip about carbohydrates is to be aware of their impact on your blood sugar level. When you eat carbohydrates the body breaks them down into glucose to be used for energy. All carbohydrates contain either slow or fast releasing sugars which effects your energy levels and can impact fat levels. Let's compare having a banana versus a bowl of porridge. Both are healthy food sources and provide good energy for the brain. However the banana contains high levels of natural sugar resulting in an energy surge followed by a plunge, whereas porridge contains low levels of sugar thus releasing energy slowly. This is why you feel hungry soon after a banana and not for a few hours after porridge. Ever notice that? So consume protein with many of your meals and fibre too. Do remember however that best to eat fruit on it's own and 30 minutes before any other foods as it digests quickly.

While I am not a fan of low/no carb nutrition plans they can play a role short term when modified from popular diets. Sometimes with clients I will get them to cut carbohydrates out of their final meal or after lunch. What this does is decrease overall calories consumed that day and then by afternoon/evening force your body to utilise more fat as fuel. Because this is not extreme your body won't go into fight or flight mode so it will burn just fat and your muscles and bones will be protected. So this can be implemented for a few weeks without any adverse effects.

So in summary carbohydrates play a crucial role in the functioning of our bodies and are wrong to be demonised. Their sole role is energy for both body and brain. While I advise you to eat a plentiful amount of them daily don't overdo it as excess may eventually store as fat if your reserves are never drawn on. Ignore no/low carbohydrate diets as they are not healthy and have many adverse effects and are not a good long term lifestyle strategy. If you are ever to decrease your daily carbohydrate intake only do so from lunchtime on to ensure that you have enough energy supply for the most active part of the day.

6 – Are All Fats Equal?

Most people believe that they should avoid all fats as fats are what make you fat. However this is not true as this generalisation has created a huge myth around fat which doesn't tell the full story. It was a few decades ago that fat become demonised in the media and such a myth was undoubtedly created to fuel the low fat food industry. Ironically following such advice is counterproductive to your goal of getting lean. Fat needs to form a percentage of your daily calorie intake but the key is consuming good fats. If you don't consume good fats then your results will be limited and you may experience some health. They are also highly beneficial for eyesight, hair and good skin.

Let me clarify about fat. Not all fats are equal. There are both good fats and bad fats. Bad fats are saturated and trans fats and are found in all confectionary, fried foods, takeaways and red meat and other animal meats to a lesser degree. Good plant based fat sources include nuts, seeds and avocados and are classified as Essential Fatty Acids(EFAs) or omega 3, 6 and 9. Your nutrition plan needs to include essential fats. The benefits are many:

- Improved memory, focus and concentration
- Bone health
- Improved general health, bodily functions and eye health

- Improved hair and skin health
- And importantly increased fat burning

As I keep stressing throughout this nutrition section losing fat and getting in shape is much more complex than just making healthier choices. There are many pieces to the jigsaw and that is why I am focused on educating you as much as I can on each nutrient so you fully understand their key role. Once you understand their role you are more likely to include them consistently and then follow a much more balanced overall nutrition plan for the rest of your life. Eating the right amount of EFAs will increase your fat burning ability. If you are not consuming adequate quantities of EFAs your fat burning gene and hormones are switched off. And when you are eating healthy balanced plant based nutrition including EFAs your fat storage genes are switched off. Make sense? So even by following a clean nutrition plan your fat burning won't reach it's full potential unless you are consuming a certain amount of EFA containing foods such as nuts, seeds and avocados.

I recommend consuming one to two portions of good fat containing foods daily. This can mean adding nut butter or avocado to a smoothie, making guacamole, having peanut butter sandwiches, having a handful of nuts and seeds or adding them to your porridge or you get a a lot of EFAs in a good muesli. There are many options but limit to one or two portions a day as remember fat is very dense calorie wise with 9 calories per gram vs 4 calories per gram for carbohydrates and protein. If you won't eat EFA containing foods then get a wholefood supplement.

Another important benefit of EFAs is keeping your joints oiled. Consistent exercise puts pressure on your joints so you must keep them healthy and lubricated. Not consuming good fats could contribute to injuries and bone problems. Start increasing your intake of essential fatty acid containing foods and start witnessing the accelerated fat loss as well as all the other great benefits I have outlined in this chapter.

7 – *Why Plant Based Makes Sense*

When my pregnant wife told me that our son was going to be raised vegan I hit the roof but knew I would have to accept it. She had her mind made up. My background in combination with my fitness/health/wellness education meant that I was totally anti vegan beliefs and customs. They seemed crazy and extreme to me and I saw them as a conspiracy theory with made up facts. I saw veganism as both a faddy diet and similar to a cult with what I saw as extreme passion in how the community shared it's message. I had just about accepted my wife going vegan about a year earlier but now my son!! This was the son I had wanted my whole life and now he was going to be vegan!! I was seriously worried. How long was it going to be until he was back in hospital with anemia or serious illness?

In this book and chapter I am not going to go deep and detailed into the last 11 years watching my son being raised vegan and personally having a 7 year journey to eventually going vegan. I am now coming up to the end of my 5th year 100% plant based. It would not be fully in keeping with the subject matter of this particular book but I do go much deeper and detailed in Go Vegan Grow which is the next book I am writing and publishing in 2017. Make sure you check that book out as it will be a must read for anyone wanting to know the truth about the main industries that run the world as well as for anyone interested in my personal journey to veganism and to find out how to successfully adopt a plant based lifestyle. This chapter will share important points in relation to why plant based nutrition is best for getting in shape and for easy maintenance and will touch on the health aspect too.

My son thrived and what I witnessed in those first 12 months both astounded and baffled me. He wasn't sick once and his development was super fast. Vegans are always sick and malnourished looking right? That was what I had been taught for years. Veganism was not a healthy diet to follow. Surely he should have been anaemic with slow growth, poor cognitive skills, regular illness etc. None of it. Nada. I was stunned. He was the healthiest most vibrant strong kid I had ever seen. It was time to question what I had learned for the previous 10 years.

And so began my research into the plant based lifestyle 11 years ago. I am not going to go too deep into everything I would like to tell you about what I have learned in the last 11 years as I am conscious that you are reading this book first and foremost because you want to get in shape. However on the other hand this book is focused on giving you the tools and strategies for regaining control over your mind/body/health and the food you eat impacts both your brain and body as well as your health so it is relevent. So in this chapter I am going to address the most important points relating to losing fat and gaining muscle. Our goal is also for you to experience abundant energy and optimal health and vitality. If you would like to learn everything I have learned about the plant based lifestyle and read my personal journey of discovery over the last 11 years make sure to grab a copy of Go Vegan Grow when it launches in 2017.

Prior to Max's birth my wife had been encouraging me to watch certain documentaries, read certain books and follow certain plant based advocates online. I ignored all of this until about 12 months after Max's birth. Like I said above what I witnessed gave me huge curiosity and I have usually fairly open minded about anything new but this one did push my boundaries largely due to the level of negativity around veganism in all I had previously learned. However I always must investigate anything proposed to improve one's mind/body/health as my personal goal has always been to experience the optimum level myself and then pass on that information to my clients. So I started watching documentaries. The more I watched and learned the more eager I was to watch more documentaries. I began reading a lot of books. I followed and spoke to many plant based advocates.

I was stunned at what I was discovering and angry about the lies I had been told my whole life but in particular I was angry about the previous 10 years when I had invested thousands in my education and mentors in my goal to be the #1 mind/body/health coach yet what I was teaching my clients was potentially hurting them long term and hindering their results. At this time I was also spending a hundred pounds a week on supplements that now turns out was damaging my body not helping it!! Read more details about supplements in Chapter 8. Now I am going to share with you the key findings of what I learned as they relate to what we are aiming to achieve with Metabolic Stimulation System.

MSS is focused on you losing fat and gaining lean muscle and getting in the best shape of your life. I also want you to experience optimal brain function and health. So how does following a plant based nutrition plan help with any of this? Let's go through the key points.

Dairy :

What I learned about dairy shocked me the most. I refer to it as the secret cause of suffering as it has a part to play in practically all suffering in terms of health conditions, pains and ailments and also for those struggling to lose fat. We are not designed to consume and break down dairy. That's right – this goes against everything we have been conditioned to believe. This is where you must keep an open mind as I aim to awaken your consciousness. You and I and the whole world have been conditioned and brainwashed by the food, dairy and supplement industries as well as by the media into thinking that we can't live without dairy. We have always been told of it's many benefits. Well the sad truth is that it is all lies. Why are we not designed to consume dairy?

Firstly it is the milk of another mammal and we are the only species on the planet that consumes another mammal's milk. This should appear strange right? But also vitally important is that in order to break down human breast milk we require 2 enzymes- rennin and latase – and after weaning age (around 2) we no longer produce these enzymes and this is when breastfeeding usually ends. So we can't even break down human breast milk so it's not going to be any different with another mammal's milk. So already on two counts we certainly are not designed to consume and break down dairy. Now why I refer to it as a secret cause of suffering is because it is only when you eliminate dairy for a period of time that you realise just how bad it is for you when you consume it again. The negative impact is immediate is mucus and breathing difficulties. You may be thinking what has this got to do with you getting visible abs – I am getting to it but I want you to understand the why remember!!

Dairy was one of the first animal based food sources I cut down on and eventually eliminated (Ben and Jerrys was the final thing I needed to let go of) in my process of gradually adopting a plant based nutrition lifestyle. We are all lactose intolerant. We can't break it down. We are not designed to. Some people show obvious symptoms early on and they are the lucky ones. For the majority they will never know that dairy is causing them harm spend years looking for reasons for their pain or health issues and also stubborn weight particularly belly fat. Dairy is highly acidic. When you consume a lot of acidic foods your body becomes very toxic and the body creates more fat cells and places them on the belly to protect the vital organs.

Your body and blood in particular must always remain alkaline or you will die. When the body is consuming acidic foods it must rebalance itself by taking calcium and other minerals from our bones. The biggest lie regarding dairy is the best calcium source and strengthens bones when it does the opposite and contributes to bone disease. How crazy is this!! This is why you need to be open minded and question anything you hear from the big industries there are many lies being told in the name of making profit.

So consuming dairy products is not helping your fat loss efforts as it's acidic nature is causing fat gain. Remember the purpose of cow's milk is to take the calf from 200 pounds at birth to 2000 pounds after 12 months or less. So like human breast milk it is for gaining size fast. Make sense? Then add the acidic nature of dairy products and the impact of this on your body and health and you should now be able to understand why it is one of the key things you need to eliminate fast. Dairy products are also high in fat mostly saturated fat. I spoke about these bad fats in the last chapter. Dairy products leech calcium from our bones. They contribute to a toxic acidic environment which leads to increased fat storage around the midsection and act as a blocker to utilising fat as a fuel source. Is this starting to make sense and sink in? Time to go dairy free. The good news is that nowadays this is easy as there is a huge range of products available. It is very different to even 10 years ago when there was very limited support of dairy free products and they tasted disgusting. In my book Go Vegan Grow I will go into great depth on my research into dairy. What I have shared in this chapter is only the tip of the iceberg.

Meat :

When I refer to meat I am referring to meat from any land based animal whether beef, chicken, pork etc. For majority of my life I have been a major meat eater. Growing up I had meat in sandwiches and dinners. At weekends I loved sunday roast. My favourite meal was lasagna. Every saturday and sunday morning I looked forward to a full fry up watching soccer am in bed. Then when I got into training and bodybuilding I took it to a whole new level in terms of my consumption.

During my 12 week programme for my Body For Life Challenge entry I was eating 13 times a day and about 7 of these included beef or turkey or chicken. Everything I had been taught about the body and training and recovery pointed towards the necessity of meat in our diets. Hence why I initially saw no logic in a plant based vegan diet. However this is where education and awareness comes in. Meat is highly acidic so, like I shared regarding dairy, this leads to many problems within the body. Acidity means toxins. Increased toxins means increased fat cells particularly as belly fat. Now of course you can say "what about bodybuilders and all the meat they eat". Remember I lived that life. You can look amazing aesthetically but internally your body can be in trouble. I experienced this through a few health wakeup calls over the years.

Our goal with MSS is not just getting in shape but creating a healthy active lifestyle remember. So we want to decrease toxicity and get our body as healthy and alkaline as possible. Another important point is that we are not designed to digest meat. Our digestive tract is too long so a lot of meat just rots inside. This is why meat is often found when people get colonic irrigations. Disgusting but true. So think about how this must be impacting how efficiently and effectively your body is operating. Remember maximum fat burning happens when your body is working at it's best. Probably the most important point I need to make is in relation to the hormones and antibiotics these animals are pumped with as they are raised before being killed. When you eat meat you are ingesting this too so it is messing up your hormone levels which has a huge impact on your fat levels. This is why so many guys are developing "man boobs" which were never evident a few decades ago. So meat is highly acidic. Meat leads to increased fat storage. Meat causes toxicity which leads to more belly fat. Meat impacts your hormone levels which has a big impact on fat levels. Am I making sense?

Fish

I am going to finish with fish. While more people have become more aware of what I have shared about meat and dairy few realise the dangers of fish which is always seen as a safe clean food to eat. However the opposite is true as most fish contain a lot of mercury. Fish has become a staple food for almost all communities across the globe but it has proven to be difficult to reduce exposure to mercury without completely avoiding fish. .Fish are contaminated with mercury through pollution caused by coal-burning factories that settles into lakes, rivers and oceans. The fish we eat absorb this mercury through a process called "bioaccumulation". This is the process through which the mercury travels from organism to organism throughout the food chain. It starts off by being absorbed by plankton, which is then eaten by crustaceans and small fish then bigger fish and then humans. A body filled with toxic substances, such as mercury, is often confined in a state of fat-loss resistance, wherein the body cannot lose fat. Until toxins are cleared from the body, individuals will struggle to lose fat, regardless of following a strict diet or exercise protocol. I have mentioned a number of times so far in this section about the negative impact of toxicity on fat loss so this just adds more weight to it. Toxins like mercury affect your hormones and create hormonal imbalances. As previously mentioned such imbalances lead to fat-loss resistance. Understanding hormones and their impact on metabolism and fat levels is critical to losing fat and getting to your "ideal" body shape. Leptin is a hormone that tells the brain to burn fat for energy. If the brain is not receiving the correct message from this hormone, due to toxic overload, then the body will not be able to burn fat for energy. What does this mean? Real and lasting fat loss is not possible when the body is in a state of toxicity, despite following a healthy nutrition and exercise regime. So I hope you can understand why eating fish is hindering your fat loss efforts and may have been doing so for years. As mentioned a few times detoxing your body is a crucial step in achieving your ideal body. No longer eating fish will be a positive step but there is something else you can do to help remove mercury from your system that has built up over years. Eat foods that contain chelating compounds. These compounds bind to the mercury in your bloodstream and remove it from the body in the form of waste. Foods that are rich in chelating compounds include:

- Brazil nuts
- Pumpkin seeds
- Cilantro
- Garlic
- Chlorella
- Turmeric

I hope what I have shared about dairy, meat and fish has given you food for thought and has made adopting a plant based lifestyle more appealing and logical. In Go Vegan Grow I will go into much more depth about everything I have addressed in this chapter as well as sharing a load more information that will shock you. I know it is a lot to take in and as a result you may even question it. What I urge you to do, as I do everyone, is to keep an open mind and do your own research and investigation into all of this. In the resources section at the back of this book I have shared details of resources I feel will help.

The benefits of following a plant based lifestyle are many. Not only do you avoid everything I have shared in this chapter but you get to eat wholefood and the food provided by nature. You get to consume food energised by the sun and you can really gain from this by consuming green based foods that contain chlorophyll such as kale, spinach, broccoli, wheatgrass etc. Now I must stress that the lifestyle I am encouraging you to follow is one that is wholefood and not processed vegan food. Whether processed food is vegan or animal based doesn't matter. It is still not good for you and leads to increasing fat levels. Another big benefit of adopting a plant based lifestyle as it is so much easier on your digestive system as you are consuming foods that the human body was designed to consume and digest. Over the next 6 weeks you will be following a plant based nutrition plan and I expect at the end of it you will be left in no doubt of the many benefits in how it will make you feel, not just in your body shape but your overall health.

8 – Supplements : Necessity Or Expensive Urine

There was a time when I was spending €120 per week on supplements. I have stated the following a few times throughout this book but this is an important learning in how industries make us think. All that i had learned in courses, read in magazines and books, heard from "experts" as well as bodybuilders and athletes I spoke with over the years pointed towards the necessity of using supplements. If you didn't use supplements then it was impossible to get the level of results you were aiming to achieve. It would be impossible to achieve a lean physique with low bodyfat levels or to become very muscular or become a faster more powerful athlete. Protein shakes were a must have. So based on what i trusted and believed I committed a sizeable chunk of my weekly income to invest in supplements. For many years I also recommended specific supplements to clients based on their goals. Being in the best shape I could be in always mattered. Being the best I could be at any endeavour always mattered. I have always been willing to take and do whatever it took, bar steroids, to achieve my goals.

My supplement experience started when I was 17. I was just getting into working out when a friend of mine's brother (who was a fitness instructor and good footballer) gave me what was left in a tub of Tony Quinn protein powder. This was good timing as from all the reading I had been doing since getting the exercise bug and from speaking to many in the gym I was starting to feel a need to start using protein shakes to maximise my gains. I used this product for a while as well as a multivitamin called Centrum which my mother had been giving me for many years. We all need multivitamins right??

A few years later after seeing an advert in a magazine I got big into Bill Phillips and his Body For Life book and Transformation Challenge which I eventually entered and won. As well as the training and nutrition there was a huge emphasis on taking supplements and even the nutrition programme included meal replacement shakes for 2 or 3 of the meals. Other products such as fat burners were also recommended. So I moved from Tony Quinn to EAS products starting with meal replacements and protein powder. I loved them. They were a huge step up in taste and from what I was reading they were a step up quality and effectiveness too. During the following years I added more EAS supplements to my supplement plan as well as trying out some other companies too My personal training business was really starting to grow at this stage so I wanted to make sure I had suitable products I trusted to recommend to clients to suit different budgets and goals.

By 2003, the year I completed my 12 week Transformation entry for the Body For Life Challenge, I was investing quite heavily in my supplements and during my 12 week training programme I was spending more on supplements than I was my food, hitting on average €120 per week. This included 2 types of protein (whey during day and casein at night just before bed and also around 3am when I would set alarm to wake up to take it -supposedly proven to be more effective than whey when asleep), meal replacement shakes, mass gainer shake, 3 types of creatine(pre workout, post workout and plain creatine monohydrate for other times during day), HMB, ZMA, multivitamin, fish oil capsules, fat burners/ thermogenics and meal replacement bars as well as protein bars. Supplements played a big part in my overall nutrition programme especially when I was consuming up to 13 meals a day. I needed to pack on a huge amount of muscle mass and defy my genetics to have a chance of winning the BFL Challenge and supplements were then a necessity weren't they? This is what I was lead to believe and what reason had I to think any other way at the time. They would hardly lie would they?

During my 12 weeks I gained 26 pounds of muscle and lost 14 pounds of fat going from 15% to 5% bodyfat in this short space of time. At the time I believed 100% that my supplement plan was a key player in my transformation and in becoming a BFL Challenge Champion but had it been? Or was it more likely down to my training and nutrition? What was the truth?

In 2004 I got into endurance sports as a new challenge and started doing 10km races and eventually marathons starting with the New York Marathon Nov 2004. I was still taking protein shakes, meal replacements and protein bars but some of the other more fat loss/bodybuilding focused supplements were gone and replaced instead with electrolyte drinks, gels and energy bars as well as glucosamine sulphate for my joint health. The multivitamin was still there too. There was no way you could get through a marathon without electrolyte drinks and gels right? This reliance on supplements was being encouraged everywhere including magazines, books, media, supermarkets and supplement stores. Every so often someone would refuse to take supplements. They were met with a shocked look of incomprehension. Were they not serious about doing the necessary for results. They needed supplements. Who was the fool?

Now let's fast track to 2016 as I write this book. My current weekly supplement expenditure is €10 tops and often would even be zero. Why? What changed? Is it that I now can't afford supplements anymore? Or did I learn something? What changed for me? Researching and studying the supplement industry was quite an eye opener. What I learned was similar to what I learned regarding the food, meat, dairy and pharmaceutical industries – profit rules over health. It was a journey quite similar to what I have shared a snippet of in the previous chapter regarding adopting a plant based lifestyle. It was a case of becoming conscious and aware of the truth about the industry. It brought the usual anger on awareness wondering why I didn't wake up to it sooner. So what changed my mind about supplements?

I would sum it up as being a combination of a few health shocks, a series of tests, a period of research and an awakening of my common sense. In the remainder of this chapter I am going to speak about synthetic supplements, wholefood supplements and what my recommendations are now for you with regard to supplements.

I want to start by clarifying what the word supplement means

**A thing added to something
else in order to complete or enhance it**
(courtesy of a google search)

So a supplement fills a gap that might be evident in our nutrition programme. So we should not have a reliance on supplements. We do not NEED supplements. If we are unwilling to consume wholefood versions of vital nutrients then we should use them to fill gaps. You have a choice. If you consume a varied wholefood plant based lifestyle you should get what you need without supplements. Let's look at two examples where one may need to invest in a supplement. Example one is if we don't eat enough fruits and vegetables then we risk the possibility of not having adequate vitamins, minerals and antioxidants. If we won't eat any good fat sources such as avocados, nuts and seeds then we run the risk of not experiencing the benefits of good fats. These 2 key nutritional areas are where many do not consume adequate amounts in wholefood form so may need to supplement.

Now the other meaning of the word supplement is "enhance it". It is this angle that the supplement industry has build it's house on and morphed "enhance" with "need" in my opinion. It is near impossible that anyone will ever be deficient in either carbohydrates or protein unless they are following some ill advised diet that is seriously calorie and nutrient deficient. In the developed world everyone consumes more than enough. Hence the obesity epidemic. From day one the supplement industry created urgency around one's protein requirements creating the impression that one needs protein shakes to get adequate protein. This is so untrue as it is near impossible not to get enough protein no matter what your eating habits are. There is protein in most foods. In addition whey protein was the lead product for these companies and whey was something that was just discarded before someone had a genius idea to use it and build a supplement industry around it.

I want to also stress that even with endurance events you will rarely need the carbohydrate supplements they recommend once you have a smart nutrition plan built around your training and races. I have been competing as a triathlete for the last 5 years and haven't taken one carbohydrate load drink or gel during either training sessions or races. I have only ever used wholefood. A balanced and varied and smart strategic nutrition plan will cover most angles. Let's take a look at each supplement category.

Vitamins & Minerals :

First let's look at vitamin and mineral supplements. The big problem with the majority of supplements is that they are synthetic. This means that they are made from chemicals in an attempt to recreate nature in various chemical compounds. Our bodies are not designed to break these chemicals down so they are either excreted in our urine (hence often dark yellow colour) or are stored in the body causing toxicity. We have spoken about the dangers of toxicity at depth in this section. What is important is that you can now see that nutrition is quite complex and that you likely have a number of areas you can work on which while frustrating should also give you hope as you now have a checklist to tick off. Isolated vitamins are not good as we are designed to consume the whole not part so consuming just the part will have no benefit and again will just become expensive urine or toxins in the body. When investing in any supplements you need to be careful to ensure that they are wholefood and have as little processing done to them as possible. More processing means less active enzymes. You are better to focus on consuming plentiful supplies of fruits, vegetables and salads and you will have no problem with a vitamin or mineral deficiency. A great way to get a huge amount of these nutrients in is via smoothies. I recommend one or two green based smoothies daily for this purpose. So my recommendation is that you don't need a multivitamin and mineral supplement but if you do decide you want one make sure it is wholefood and natural. Also don't waste your money on isolated vitamins or minerals.

Protein :

Now let's discuss the supplement industry's golden child – protein. The industry was born out of protein shakes and whey protein in particular. Where did whey come from? It came from part of the milk that had always been discarded. Then someone had the genius idea of using it for cheap food and then to make Whey Protein shakes. Add a convincing script to it about needing more protein and now trillions are spent annually by people fearful of a protein deficiency when it is practically impossible. Every food source contains a level of protein and our requirement daily is about 10% of total calorie intake. This is so much less than recommended. No one should have difficulty meeting their protein requirement daily so protein shakes are totally unnecessary. If you are very active you will have an extra requirement for protein as you will with all nutrients but it will be nowhere near the level the supplement industry would have you believe. Protein shakes used to be a core part of my nutrition plan but now I rarely use them instead using wholefood.

When I did a 6 month experiment without having protein shakes and just eating food I expected to lose a lot of muscle and see my performance and results suffer but it never happened. I do still occasionally add some wholefood plant based protein powder to my smoothies. This is usually during periods of heavy training volume. Also I may use it if I don't fancy other protein wholefood sources. The brands I would recommend are Vega and Sun Warrior. Protein shakes and meal replacements are no longer something I use on a daily basis. I now much prefer wholefood smoothies with avocados or nuts/nut butters as my protein source.

Carbohydrates :

What about carbohydrate supplements like electrolyte drinks and gels? Now for the topic of this book this is not hugely relevant but it will possibly be for your goals once you have achieved your transformation. I have seen many clients decide to do a 10km, marathon or even a triathlon after they have achieved their ideal body. Humans are designed for growth and challenge so you should always be striving for something. These carbohydrate products are promoted on the basis of needing a carbohydrate/ sugar/glucose boost during a training session or a race. However when you have carb loaded or just eaten a normal day's food your muscles glycogen stores will most likely be adequate and if they run out there will be some stored glycogen in your liver and if that runs out then your body will turn to fat as fuel. So even without electrolyte drinks and gels there should be enough glycogen to get you through most races of a certain distance when exercising for about 60 mins to 90 minutes. For longer races such as marathon or ultras or olympic distance triathlon and longer triathlon distances it would provide a boost if more carbohydrates were ingested during the session. Personally I prefer to now use wholefood forms like raw bars, dates or occasionally wholefood plant based shakes. I would not advise using the pure sugar supplements like gels and drinks as while they will provide immediate energy this will also lead to a dramatic fall in energy soon after with a need for a further kick of glycogen. So I do not recommend any of these carbohydrate drinks, bars and gels.

EFAs :

Next let's look at EFAs – Essential Fatty Acids. Before going plant based vegan I spent many years using fish oil capsules as well as oils such as Udo's Oil to ensure I was getting enough EFAs. I have read much information over the years of the many benefits of adding this supplement including healthier hair, skin and nails. Also better brain function and eyesight and very relevant to this book's topic – increased fat burning. Now since going plant based vegan Jan 1st 2012 I have not used any EFAs supplement despite there being vegan EFAs on the market. And being honest I have not felt that my body has missed them in any way. Now I am not saying they are not beneficial. Just that not consuming one hasn't made much difference to me. I get adequate EFAs via avocados, nuts and nut butters and this shows by not needing a supplement. However this is one supplement I would recommend for most people as most don't consume enough EFA containing foods. The product I would recommend is Udo's Oil. I'll repeat that consuming a very varied and balanced nutrition plan usually covers all requirements.

B12 :

Finally I want to address vitamin B12 as you are going to be following a plant based lifestyle for 6 weeks. Debate surrounding Vitamin B12 regularly pops up. Meat eaters claim that vegans have to be deficient in B12 as you can only get it from meat. However I have had many clients get B12 assessments and their results have blown doctors away who have not been able to understand their levels. It comes down again to eating a varied balanced plan. Vegan sources of B12 are foods fortified with B12 (including some plant milks, some soy products and some breakfast cereals) and B12 supplements. There is also the option of getting B12 shots. I recommend clients to get their B12 levels checked a couple of times a year and also to either get occasional B12 shot or use a B12 supplement like I do. I use a liquid form that you put under your tongue for maximum absorption. I only occasionally use it and more as an insurance policy versus feeling I need it. We use Solgar brand. If your B12 levels are low you will know as your energy will be seriously low.

So that covers the main supplement categories. I hope what I have shared has made sense and you now look on supplements and the industry very differently. I am regularly approached by supplement companies looking to sponsor me products so if products look good I will give them a trial and then report how I find them. So keep eye on my social media in particular where I share this information. Make sure to check out any supplements you may consider using and make sure they are wholefood based created by ethical companies. Remember a wholefood plant based nutrition plan will cover most bases once it is varied and balanced.

Next we get into your MSS Nutrition programme.

9 – Your MSS Nutrition Programme

Now that you should understand the theoretical side of a healthy balanced nutrition plan it is now time to piece it all together into your MSS Nutrition programme for the next 6 weeks. Following this programme should set the foundation for a life of feeding your body what it needs and should also eliminate cravings for foods that serve no positive purpose in your body.

See below lists of foods for each food source that you can choose from in designing your daily nutrition plan. There may be some left out that you like to use. The main purpose of the following list is to give you a shopping list but if you want to add anything that is fine once it is wholefood and falls into the type of foods I have recommended in the book so far.

Carbohydrates :

- white potatoes(occasional)
- sweet potatoes (preferred)
- pasta (spelt #1, wholewheat #2)
- rice (basmati #1, wholemeal #2, white #3)
- couscous (brown #1 white #2)
- Fajita/burrito wraps – tortilla wraps
- Quinoa (high protein content but going to classify here as a carb choice as grain part of meal)
- Noodles

- Bread (Spelt #1 Oat #2 wholemeal/wholegrain #3)
- Wholemeal pitta breads/pockets (no white allowed)
- Fruit – any fruit is allowed as all good for you
- Porridge oats
- Muesli – 100% natural one with no added sugars and sweeteners
- Oat Cakes
- Rice Cakes

Protein :

- Chickpeas
- Lentils
- Kidney beans
- Butter beans
- Canneloni beans
- Any other type of beans
- Tofu
- Seitan
- Any Nut butters (no salt or sugar)
- Any Nuts (in their original state)
- Any Seeds
- Avocados
- Sunwarrior Protein Powder
- Vega Protein Powder

Fats :

- Avocados
- Any Nuts (original state)
- Any Nut butters (no salt or sugar)
- Any Seeds

- Olive or coconut oil (use sparingly – mindful 9 calories per gram)

Vegetables & Salad :

- All are allowed – there is no such thing as a bad one unless not in natural state

Other :

- Soya Milk
- Rice Milk
- Almond Milk
- Oat Milk
- Dairy free Yoghurt- can be soya, rice, coconut
- Nakd bars
- Trek bars
- Flour (brown or spelt preferred – white occasionally)
- Tomato Puree
- Herbs – any are good to use
- Sea salt
- Vegetable stock cubes
- Green tea

The list of carbohydrate options includes only slow-release carbohydrates (except fruit) and mostly unprocessed as during the 6 weeks we must minimise any insulin spikes and want to maintain stable blood sugar levels throughout. The protein choices are all vegan as I have recommended that you follow a 100% plant based vegan nutrition plan for the 6 weeks. If you are adamant that you don't want to follow a plant based nutrition plan during the next 6 weeks then substitute any of the plant based protein sources with an animal based source. But in making this decision be mindful of what I shared in Chapter 7 about meat and dairy's impact on your fat levels and results and also importantly your health. Being 100% plant based with your nutrition will ensure you achieve the best results and will also allow you to experience the difference in being 100% plant based vs the alternative. Once the 6 weeks ends the choice is yours. Now I cannot force you to follow my advice for the next 6 weeks but I do hope that what I shared in Chapter 7 has got your thinking and looking at food differently. I hope it has opened up your mind to plant based nutrition.

While I recommend that you include good fat containing foods each day be sure to only have 2 portions a day maximum. Remember that each gram of fat has over double the calories of both carbohydrates and protein (9 calories vs 4 calories per gram). Eat as much vegetables and salad as you can fit in during each day. These foods along with fruit need to be a key foundation of your nutrition plan as I repeated during this book. Eating high fibre foods like these also means that you will feel satisfied after eating a large quantity. You will then be more likely to control your portions of carbohydrates and protein in your meals. Make sure to eat a wide variety of vegetables and salad as there are so many choices and they all have individual benefits.

Here are the rules for your MSS nutrition programme:

- Have breakfast 15 minutes after rehydrating first thing in the morning or eat 30 to 60 minutes after training session if exercising first thing in the morning.

- Eat small balanced meals every 3 hours – carbohydrates, protein and vegetables/salad each meal and a portion of fats with one or two of the meals/snacks
- Your portion guidelines are as follows : ¼ plate carbohydrates, ¼ plate protein and ½ plate vegetables and salad. Eat more vegetables and salad should you wish.
- Don't eat within 4 hours of bed
- Drink 4 litres of water (up to 6 litres if able) each day starting with 1 litre first thing each morning. Work towards 4 litres using water protocol outlined in Chapter 1 if you are currently drinking less than 4 litres daily.

When designing your daily MSS nutrition programme and meal/snack timings it is important to consider the following :

- Waking time
- Bedtime
- Training time
- Hours of work
- Breaks allowed
- When you need to prepare meals and when you can cook at home
- When you must eat out whether for business, pleasure, convenience or social

Make sure you vary your choices for each food source. This will be important to avoid boredom. Also every food source has different nutrients so variety is important so that you get as much variety as possible in all nutrient types.

It is very important that you take the time to review and plan at the end of each day. Make sure to keep a food diary. Use the MSS nutrition logger you can access in the resources section. Please take time each night to plan the following day and prepare meals/snacks where necessary to bring with you. Each night you should fill in what you actually ate compared to what you had planned. Sometimes it can be different due to unexpected circumstances. This way you will be able to see how well you are doing as well as identifying trends and focusing on where you may need to tweak your plan. Having a plan is great but often you will need to go to plan B. Life tends to have a habit of keeping us on our toes.

See a sample diary entry of planned v actual below. Use this as a guideline for planning your daily nutrition plan. Also don't forget to access your MSS nutrition plan logger in the resources page at the back of the book and fill it in at the end of each day. This will be an invaluable tool for you. Remember to use it to review and plan – key to success. There will also be details of how you can access many plant based recipes that will give you ideas for the next 6 weeks and beyond.

Planned V Actual Example :

Planned :

Actual :

Meal 1 :
7am Porridge, raisins,
banana, linseeds, walnuts

Meal 1 :
7.15am Porridge, raisins,
banana, linseeds, walnuts

Meal 2 :
10am Fruit salad of
Mixed fruits homemade
(not shop bought) with
soya natural yoghurt
and flaxseeds

Meal 2 :
10.30am Choc Loco Nakd
bar due to unexpected
meeting

Meal 3 :
1pm salad of lettuce,
spinach, broccoli,
cucumber, tomato,
onion, beetroot, tofu
avocado with 2 slices
oat bread and hummus

Meal 3 :
1pm Salad of lettuce,
spinach, broccoli,
cucumber, tomato,
onion, beetroot, tofu
avocado, with 2 slices
oat bread and hummus

Meal 4 :
4pm Handful almonds
and some grapes

Meal 4 :
4.10pm Trek choc bar

Meal 5 :
7pm Chickpea curry
with basmati rice and
homemade spicy wedges

Meal 5 :
7.30pm Chickpea curry
with basmati rice and
homemade spicy wedges

Can you see above where there were times a few
tweaks had to be made and Plan B implemented due to
unexpected situations? The key is being prepared so

always have quick and easy snacks like fruit, nuts, seeds, trek and nakd bars, smoothies etc with you wherever you go as well as always having a bottle water with you.

You can access our plant based recipe book packed with delicious recipes we use ourselves by going to the link indicated in the resources section at the back of this book.

You have now been educated in "lifelong" nutritional strategies and you should now have a better understanding of the importance of both macro and micro nutrients. You have been given the MSS nutrition plan guidelines and can access many balanced delicious plant based recipes in the resources section at the back of the book. What you must do is each evening take time to plan out your nutrition for the following day using the macro and micro nutrients authorised food lists. Then prepare what you need in advance and you will be all set. Create your personalised daily nutrition programme based on your own lifestyle, working demands and daily commitments using the shopping list and recommended recipes provided. I have even included the MSS nutrition logger in the resources section.

What matters now is following the programme guidelines. This is important in achieving your best results. It works! It has already been proven with hundreds of clients around the world in the last few years. Remember too that nutrition plays 80% role in your results. Within 6 weeks you will have regained control of your mind/body/health and will be in the best shape of your life. And most importantly you will have lived a healthy active lifestyle for 6 weeks. This lifestyle will be easily maintained for the rest of your life. Gone are the days of diets and deprivation. Gone are the days of ineffective exercise and hours in the gym wasting your time, energy and money. An exciting future awaits. The new you awaits. Get excited and start taking action now.

The recipe book you will get access to in the resources section will include ideas for :

Breakfast suggestions
Lunch Suggestions
Dinner Suggestions
Snack Suggestions

Section 4 : Sleep

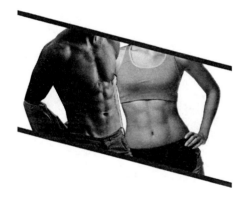

1 – How Much Sleep Is Enough?

In the previous three sections I have taught you everything you need to know about

1. Creating a positive focused mindset
2. Effective Metabolic Stimulation training methods and
3. Healthy balanced wholefood plant based nutrition.

Each of these play a crucial role in our MSS formula in successfully transforming your mind/body/health. These 3 areas are crucial to your transformation and long term lifestyle change. However these are only 3 of the 4 crucial parts of the formula in achieving your desired outcome. Before reading this book I am sure that you understood to some degree that exercise and nutrition played an important role in achieving results. Hopefully now you have a much clearing understanding of why certain fat loss and body transformation methods work, as well as why certain ones don't. In the last few years I have been glad to see that a growing number of people are starting to realise the key role mindset plays in success. However most people are totally unaware of how important a role getting quality sleep plays on not just your results but every aspect of your life. Without quality sleep results will be minimal and life in general will be challenging!!

Are you always tired and lethargic despite 8-12 hours sleep each night? Do you get the afternoon slump? Do you find it difficult to get to sleep? Do you wake frequently at night? In this section I will educate you thoroughly about sleep as well as sharing our MSS sleep protocol which when implemented and followed will transform your sleep, energy and results.

Think about how you feel and act when you are tired. And poor quality sleep plays havoc with your hormones and leads to fat storage. Sleep is an area I have studied for many years now and I was initially shocked at how big an impact it plays on all areas of life. For the purposes of this book I will be focusing on it's impact on decreasing fat levels and positively impacting your metabolism. Our goal with MSS is to transform your body shape and gain control over your mind/body/health. You can read much more about sleep's impact on all areas of your life in my other book coming in 2017 - Formula 4 Success.

The period of time you spend sleeping is actually the most important of your day. It is when your training efforts and adherence to a healthy balanced nutrition program reap their rewards. It is while you sleep that the body goes to work. It is during this time that your body's sole focus is on repairing and rejuvenating and adapting to the impact of what happened during the day. If you don't experience high-quality and a suitable quantity of sleeping hours your recovery will be minimal. This will have a big impact on your results. Mindset training creates that positive mental environment where you believe you are going to achieve. Exercise breaks down the muscle fibres, and nutrition feeds the body with key nutrients to recover. Sleep is the crucial final piece. It is the part of your day that allows your body the chance to recover and use nutrients to recover and repair those microfibre tears. As previously stressed sleep may be the final piece of the 4 part formula but it is crucial as without quality sleep results will be minimal and all your efforts with mind/exercise/nutrition will not be taken advantage of.

Sleep is the only time of the day that you are totally inactive. It is the only time your body is totally at rest and recuperating. However just getting sleep is not enough. While there is an optimum quantity of sleep that is recommended what is more important is that your sleep is of sufficient quality. The quantity vs quality rule applies to most things in life. Too much focus is continuously placed on the quantity of sleep people get in this fast paced world. People are always complaining that they don't get enough sleep and feel tired and lethargic continuously. Many still feel tired after getting 10 or 12 hours sleep at the weekend when attempting to catch up. On that note I want to let you know that catching up is not possible. Why such people continuously feel tired no matter what they do is a result of poor sleep quality. Without taking the right steps sleep quantity becomes insignificant and has no positive impact no matter how long. Throughout this book you have read about the importance of quality over quantity in all aspects.

I believe and now know with certainty, from extensive research as well as experimenting on myself, that too much sleep is actually worse for you than too little. Also too little sleep is damaging to your overall health too. This is an area I have done a 360 on my opinion and in what I teach my clients. Up to 2010 when I wrote "6 Weeks To A Cover Model Body" I was totally wrong in what I believed was an "optimum" sleeping pattern. I was wrong in the advice I was giving to clients as well as in that book. For over 12 years I believed that 5 or 6 hours of sleep was adequate. I nearly saw it as a badge of honour that I could get by with so little sleep which gave me more hours than most each day to get more done. I used to jokingly(although half serious) say that sleep was a waste of time and that we only need a few hours. However this was based on years of low quantity (and quality I found out around this time) sleep when I ran my chain of fitness centres and fitness businesses. Sleep was at the bottom of my priorities. However I thought I felt fine and that I was getting more than enough sleep.

My sleeping habits and how I felt each day had just become the "norm" and because I felt ok I thought I was getting enough sleep. This is the problem. Both positively and negatively our bodies are amazing in their ability to adapt to any stimulus whether good or bad. This does not always lead to a positive outcome! My body had just adapted to what I was forcing it to do. It realised 5 or 6 hours was the most sleep I was going to get and just got on with the job of adapting to this to create a "norm". The problem was that contrary to what I believed I was not operating at my highest mental or physical potential. It was impossible to. Too little sleep over a prolonged period of time will have serious health consequences especially in the brain where it has been proven that holes can appear. Years of poor sleep, in both quality and quantity, came back to bite a few times with some scary experiences. This forced me into dedicating time to extensively research sleep and find out what the truth was about optimal sleep. For 12 years I had been seriously sleep deprived. After adjusting my sleeping routine following my in-depth research into sleep the difference was phenomenal. I will be sharing the exact strategies I use in my own life now in the next chapter.

Now let's look at those getting loads of sleep. Most people sleep anywhere from 6 to 12 hours per night but still remain tired and lethargic throughout each day. And most people sleep longer at weekends. The more sleep they get the more tired they feel. What this illustrates without any doubt is low-quality sleep. So, if you are one of those people who always feels tired despite getting 8 to 12 hour sleep you must address the quality of your sleep. That is the issue not the quantity. The next chapter will explain exactly step by step what you need to do to rectify this situation.

So the lesson to learn from this chapter is that you can sleep too little or too much. There is a certain level of sleep that you need. In the next chapter, I will reveal my protocol for experiencing high-quality sleep every night and even in situations where you may only be able to get 3 or 4 hours sleep. You will still wake up fresh and wide awake and alert ready for the day ahead. It is important to have a full understanding about how sleep works and how to get optimal sleep in every situation as there will be times you can get recommended sleep quantity as well as occasions where you can only get a few hours sleep.

2 – How to Sleep Like A Baby Every Night

In the previous chapter I stressed the important role sleep plays not even in our ability to burn fat and get in better shape but on our whole life. And I hope it has sunk in now that there needs to be a particular focus on experiencing high quality sleep every night. In that chapter I admitted how I was totally wrong for over a decade in what I practiced and preached about effective sleeping habits. This chapter will continue to educate you about aspects of sleep as well as giving you the exact protocol and step by step plan to experience high quality sleep every night. I promise you that when you implement what I teach you in this chapter you won't even need an alarm clock (will just have one set to be safe). You will wake up each morning alert, fresh and ready for action. These strategies I am about to share with you are powerful and 9 times out of 10 my clients experience better sleep on their first night implementing them. How does that sound?

There are 3 main areas we need to address and make changes in :

1. Your association with the bedroom
2. Your Sleeping Environment
3. Your Pre Sleep activities

I am going to now address each one. I will explain why each is important and then give you the steps to follow to improve on them. Your job will be to implement the steps. Remember knowledge is not power, taking action and implementing knowledge is!!

Area 1 : Your association with the bedroom

First we'll start with your association with the bedroom. What do I mean by this? What I mean is subconsciously what activity or activities does your mind subconsciously expect as you head towards and into the bedroom. What thoughts and expectations are triggered. This is so much more important than you or most of the world realise. You need to associate your bedroom with sleep first and foremost and we'll throw in sex too. But let's stay focused here. Let's focus on creating a positive association with the bedroom towards sleep. You need this association embedded in your subconscious so that it is triggered as you go to enter your bedroom. How do you do that? Pay attention to what I am about to say.

If you watch tv in the bedroom or work in the bedroom or study in the bedroom or spend hours on social media in the bedroom then your mind associates the bedroom with these activities. You must destroy these associations and create positive ones in relation to getting quality sleep. You need to create positive associations as mentally you will trigger certain expectations when you enter the bedroom. When you enter the bedroom, you want your mind to think "this is the time to go to sleep, time to rest, time to relax" so I better start releasing melatonin – the hormone for sleepiness. You need to be able to wind down your body and mind so that you go to bed in a very relaxed and peaceful state. If your subconscious associates anything but sleep with the bedroom you will struggle to relax your mind, release little melatonin and struggle to get to sleep and experience quality sleep.

So you need to change your activities if you do any of the above or similar in the bedroom. Do them somewhere else and create associations there. For example work should be done in the office (home or outside of home) not in bedroom or kitchen or sitting/dining room. The next area ties into this one.

Area 2 : Your Sleeping Environment

So area 1 was about creating a positive association with the bedroom. So if you subconsciously get in the right frame of mind you have made a positive step but it doesn't stop there re the bedroom. There is a lot more action you need to take in particular relating to the actual sleeping environment i.e. what is actually in your bedroom and what it is like there. An important first step is creating a bat cave. What I mean by this is that the room is pitch dark when you switch off light to go to sleep. You do this using blackout curtains or blinds, curtains or a combination. Why is this necessary? We naturally react to light and dark. When it's dark you feel sleepier. When it's bright you feel more alive and awake. Correct? To clearly illustrate this so you fully understand it I am going to use the following two scenarios comparing how you feel during the summer and winter. In the summertime when it is brighter in the mornings we tend to wake up earlier. Right? This is assuming you haven't created your batcave yet! Waking up earlier just naturally happens without intention. Also during the summer we feel wide awake at 10pm or later when it's still bright. Take an example of having a BBQ with some friends in your garden. It could be 11pm and you still don't feel tired – correct? Now let's look at the opposite scenario. It's wintertime when it gets bright about 8.30am and dark at about 4.30pm. It's mostly dark and cold, windy and miserable. How do you feel these mornings? or even at 6pm at night? Or even at 4.30pm when it is starting to get dark? Tired and lethargic right? It's the total opposite of how you feel during the same time of the day in the summer. When it's dark people naturally feel sleepier, lethargic and find it difficult to get up in the mornings. They also get tired earlier in the evening. Can you relate to this? Is this describing you? Does my statement "we react to light and dark" make sense now? So this is why we need to create a batcave so that we have the right environment light wise when we want or need to go to bed. This will stimulate melatonin release and will be important as one of the key steps in ensuring good quality sleep.

Next it is important to wear comfortable bed clothes, not too heavy, not too light. You don't want to be too cold or hot. Our objective is creating a sleeping environment which is relaxing, peaceful and comfortable for you. You also want to have a good quality mattress. You will spend a minimum of ⅓ of your life in bed sleeping so this is a worthwhile investment and should be a no brainer really. Invest in quality and you will also have it for years.

Next let's look at what is in the bedroom. Do you have a tv? Laptop? Mobile phone? Electric alarm clock?

You need to ensure that you don't have any electrical equipment in your room. This means no tv, electric alarm clocks, clock radios and definitely no mobile phone. Even if on standby such items will transmit radiation into your sleeping environment preventing your mind shutting down. Your vessel will look asleep but your mind won't be as it will be continuously stimulated by these devices. The phone is the biggest culprit as most use it as an alarm, have their notifications turned on so pings every time there is a new one(burst of radiation each time even if on silent) and usually have their phone charging by their head!! Instead of your mobile phone or electric clock radio use a battery alarm clock. If you really do want to have your phone on at night in case of some emergency then leave it outside your door. You will still hear it but won't have the negative impact on your sleep by having it by your head or even in your room. Make sure all electrical items are plugged out so there will be no radiation or electricity around keeping you mentally awake. Make sure to start making these changes tonight!

Area 3 : Your Pre Sleep Activities

Up to this point we have discussed creating a positive association with the bedroom as well as a peaceful and suitable sleeping environment within the bedroom. Now we must focus on your pre-sleep activities which ultimately determine the quality of your sleep. If you have been watching TV, surfing the net, exercising, finishing projects for work, using your laptop, studying, drinking coffee or any such activities before bed you will not experience quality sleep. It is imperative that you shut down and relax your brain before sleep. Otherwise you will remain mentally alert, even though physically shattered and sleepy. You must take time before bed to totally relax your mind and leave the day behind you. For a minimum of 30 minutes before bed avoid TVs, computers, work, exercise or anything stimulating to your mind. Although used as a means of relaxation, watching TV stimulates your brain due to the rays being transmitted from it. The same applies to computers, mobile phones and any electrical device. You may fall asleep watching TV but mentally you are still awake.

For 30 minutes before bed choose one or more of the following to wind down:

- Have a bath or shower
- Listen to soothing, calm music
- Meditate or do some stretching, yoga or pilates
- Read fiction or non work related material that doesn't stimulate your thinking and ideas
- Relaxation or breathing techniques

Even by spending 10 minutes before bed enjoying such activities you will notice a huge difference in the quality of your sleep as you will then go to bed in a relaxed mental and physical state. It's all about creating a routine with your sleep and prioritising what you need to do. I will stress it again – you must experience quality deep sleep in order to be fully rested and wake up alert and ready the next morning.

Your Personal Sleep Cycle

I want to start by shattering the myth that you can catch up on your sleep as many do at weekends. It is impossible to catch up. Once it is gone it is gone. You must focus on the next day and getting yourself back into a sleep cycle and routine as I will explain in this section. You can't catch up but you could add another full sleep cycle some days and feel better for it. The more cycles you experience the better. I'll explain more about understanding your personal sleep cycle in this section. Everyone has and needs a sleeping rhythm/cycle. Erratic and irregular quantities of sleep added to irregular waking and bedtimes will leave you in a state of feeling permanently tired and lethargic. This has a detrimental effect on both your ability to lose fat and build lean muscle. It will mess up your hormones which are so crucial to repair. Growth hormone is released at night-time especially in the first part of the night. And due to lack of sleep the release of cortisol will increase your chances of actually gaining fat!!

Do you work on shifts? Shift work has a major impact on sleeping patterns but can be counteracted with careful planning and structuring of your day. All obstacles can be overcome. It is crucial for shift workers to follow my tips in the 3 areas of association, sleeping environment and pre sleep activities as you are looking to fool your brain into thinking it is night-time even though you will often be going to bed in the morning or during the day. While I am referring to shift workers each day you have a waking time (starting point) and a bedtime (endpoint). Structure your daily routine from your waking time, whether that is 12pm, 5pm or 6 am and stick to the guidelines outlined in section 3 in terms of your nutrition schedule for the day. This was a bit of a tangent but important to add this in for anyone dealing with shift work.

So how much sleep is actually enough? For most it is between 7 and 9 hours with 8 to 9 being the optimum. However every one of us has a specific individual sleep cycle which can vary between 1 hr 15 mins and 1 hr 45 mins in duration. Your sleep cycle is the period from when you are in light sleep then go through the various stages of sleep up until REM (Rapid Eye Movement) phase of sleep which is the deepest stage of sleep and then you come back out to light sleep and repeat. You MUST hit REM sleep a few times each night to feel rested and alert each morning. REM is when the body is recovering and repairing. Those who don't address the 3 areas I spoke of earlier will rarely if ever reach REM stage of sleep and thus will always feel tired and lethargic. So make sure to implement the steps I taught you about the 3 areas. Your personal sleep cycle has a bearing on how many hours you should aim to sleep each night. Personally my sleep cycle is 1 hr 45 minutes. How do I know this? As part of my in-depth research into sleep I tested myself to find out my personal sleep cycle. I did this by noting the time and how I felt during the night when I both unintentionally and intentionally woke up. For a period of 3 months I set alarms at various intervals after I went to sleep. I wanted to test how I felt after 1 hour or 2 hours or 3 and ½ hours.

NOTE – this was all after ensuring I covered all the steps of the 3 areas as that is crucial.

I was then able to see trends as to how I felt waking up after a certain duration of sleep. I also noted my bed times and final waking times and how I felt. From this information I was able to deduce that my personal sleep cycle was in or around 1 hr 45 mins. So this means that if I get 3 sleep cycles in the night (3 x 1 hr 45 mins = 5 hrs 15 mins) I am better off than if I got 6 hours sleep as I would be waking up in the middle of a cycle in a deep phase of sleep. Same applies that I would be better off getting 8 hr 45 mins sleep (5 x 1 hr 45 mins) than 8 hrs sleep which again would be in the middle of a cycle. Does that make sense? Now I am not telling you have to go the extent I did to find out my sleep cycle. For most it is around 1 hr 30 mins so use that as your guide. Which means you need to get 3, 4 and ½, 6 or 7 and ½ hours sleep or at most 9 hours. This is so important and without respecting your personal sleep cycle you will feel the ill effects. So based on your sleep cycle make a judgement on when your bed and waking time should be. Do your best to create a set routine of for example going to bed at 11pm and waking up then at 6.30am or 8am. Routine is very important. The number of hours of sleep that you get each night must be consistent. However it is ok if you only get 3 or 4 sleep cycles in a few nights once it is not becoming a trend. You need between 7 and 9 hours sleep each night to perform at your optimum level. Your fat levels, lean muscle levels, energy and alertness are relying on this. This final piece of the jigsaw determines your level of results.

Alcohol and Sleep :

You may not like to hear this but alcohol sabotages quality sleep even if you have implemented everything i have taught you so far. If you drink alcohol your mind does not rest despite you physically appearing asleep. Alcohol prevents you reaching the rapid eye movement phase of sleep which I spoke of in a previous paragraph. It is the deepest and most critical sleep stage for muscle recovery. As I have explained your sleeping pattern goes in cycles from light sleep, to medium sleep, to deep sleep and back to light sleep again. It is very important that you experience a number of periods of deep sleep during your sleeping cycle in order to wake up rejuvenated and refreshed and to allow your body to repair. With alcohol in your system you are ensuring this does not happen.

Now I am not expecting you to never drink alcohol again but it is important you understand alcohol's impact. Before reading this section your sleep quality was likely very poor. At least now you know of many steps you can take to improve it. Don't let alcohol ruin this. However if you have a night out or a few drinks at home just ensure that you tick as many boxes as possible to have the best sleep possible. What I would like you to do and I recommend is that for the next 6 weeks you eliminate alcohol completely. Success means sacrifice.

Stress and Sleep :

Stress has become a huge part of modern life and is another reason why the pre sleep relax and unwind session is crucial. Regardless of what is going on in your life, no matter how stressful things are, you need to shut down. If you are going to bed still focused on stressful situations and full of worry you will guarantee poor sleep. Your mind will be unable to shut down and you will almost certainly experience restless sleep too. Do your best to control your stress levels. However I appreciate this is easier said than done. I have experienced much stress at various times in my life and even though I know the theory sometimes it is just near impossible to switch off and slow down the mind. What i'd advise is that if stressed take time out each night for an activity you love and that you find relaxing.

Journalling and Gratitude :

Journalling is an activity I do each night and one that I strongly recommend you do too. It is a way of finishing off the day on a positive note which will play a key role in relaxing your mind just before you go into your pre sleep activities. I recommend that you reflect on your day and write a few notes about how it went including 3 things you are grateful for that day as well as 3 successes you had – big or small. There is always so much we have to be grateful for but we fail to see it in this fast paced world. And even in the worst of days we always have successes but again we are all too focused on what we didn't get done and what is yet to do and the next project/challenge instead of celebrating what we achieved today. These 2 activities as part of a journalling habit will be a great start to your pre sleep routine.

Your MSS Sleep Protocol :

So that was a lot of information to take in but I hope it has all made sense to you. I believe in educating people on the why before telling them what they need to do. Adherence is far more likely then and we are looking at creating a lifestyle. Here is our MSS sleep protocol for achieving a relaxed, peaceful and positive state ensuring pleasant dreams. Each night before bed do the following :

- Think about your goals
- Read or think about your why list
- Read or visualise your success scene

By using this strategy you will fall asleep relaxed and in a positive state. Your dreams will tend to incorporate whatever was foremost on your mind just prior to sleep. Hence the reason you have the types of dreams you do when stressed and worried. By following my strategy your goals will come to life in your dreams and this will create more belief in your subconscious with regarding your goal. With my strategy you will live your future through your dreams. This will reinforce your belief that achieving your goals is only a matter of taking consistent action and time. Remember how much I stressed the power of belief and visualisation in Section 1? Does this make sense to you?

So in summary if you want to sleep like a baby experiencing high-quality sleep every night:

- Create a positive association with the bedroom with sleep
- Create a bat cave
- Wear comfortable loose fitting clothes and invest in a good mattress
- Take out all electrical equipment from your room or if going to have it there unplug it all
- Journal before bed including gratitudes and successes
- Choose relaxing pre sleep activities
- Avoid alcohol before bed
- Leave stress and worry for tomorrow before you sleep

- Create positive feelings by reading your goals, whys, success scene and visualise your future

By following what I have outlined in this section you will see a dramatic difference in your sleeping patterns and experience the knock on effect during each day. You will feel invigorated and rejuvenated and you will have completed the final part of the 4 piece formula for achieving maximum results. Over the course of the next 6 weeks you mind/body/health and life will be transformed – Enjoy the journey.

Resources

I really hope that this book has been of tremendous value to you so far and that I delivered on my promise that it would be the most comprehensive step by step blueprint for regaining control over your mind/body/health.

My goal in writing Metabolic Stimulation System was to provide you with an education and understanding of the 4 key areas – mindset, exercise, nutrition and sleep. If you understand these areas and you understand why I am recommending you take a certain action you are more likely to take it – does that make sense?

This section will provide you with some resources that you can use in following the 6 week programme. Also make sure to check out the resources webpage at: www.metabolicstimulationsystem.com/resources

If you have not already been added to our private MSS Facebook Group then send a join request at https://www.facebook.com/groups/130987263732435

Should you have any questions about anything in this book feel free to contact us on one of the following:

Email : dave@dave-sheahan.com

Facebook: https://www.facebook.com/DaveSheahanPage/

Twitter: https://twitter.com/davesheahan1

Instagram: http://www.instagram.com/davesheahan1978

Snapchat : username is davesheahan

I would also love to hear your feedback on this book and would greatly appreciate if you would recommend it to others should you feel they need to read it.

Goal Statement

Write out your goal statement below making sure it is

1. Clearly defined
2. Measurement
3. Unrealistic in the perception of others

My Whys

List out your whys in relation to your goal statement on the following 2 pages. Just let your whys flow and focus mainly on what positives will come into your life on achieving your goal.

1.

2.

3.

4.

5.

6.

7.

8.

9.

10.

11.

12.

13.

14.

15.

16.

17.

18.

19.

20.

21.

22.

23.

24.

25.

26.

27.

28.

29.

30.

31.

32.

33.

34.

35.

36.

37.

38.

39.

40.

41.

42.

43.

44.

45.

46.

47.

48.

49.

50.

My Success Scene

Your Success Scene should expand on your goal statement and be treated like a script for a seconds of your personal movie scene if there was one illustrating your success. Incorporate all of your senses and where relevent any of your whys. Write your success scene in the present tense on the rest of this page and the next one if needed. The more detailed your success scene is the more vivid your visualisation sessions will be as you visualise this moment.

My MSS Journey in Photos

Photos are one of the most powerful progress measures you can use so please use the next 21 pages to track your 6 week MSS journey in photos.

Day 1 Front View Photo   Date: /   /

Day 1 Side View Photo   Date: /   /

Day 1 Side Back Photo   Date: /   /

Day 7 Front View Photo   Date: /   /

Day 7 Side View Photo   Date: /   /

Day 7 Back View Photo   Date: /   /

Day 14 Front View Photo   Date: /   /

Day 14 Side View Photo   Date: /   /

Day 14 Back View Photo   Date: /   /

Day 21 Front View Photo   Date: /   /

Day 21 Side View Photo   Date: /   /

Day 21 Back View Photo   Date: /   /

Day 28 Front View Photo   Date: /   /

Day 28 Side View Photo   Date: /   /

Day 28 Back View Photo   Date: /   /

Day 35 Front View Photo   Date: /   /

Day 35 Side View Photo   Date: /   /

Day 35 Back View Photo   Date: /   /

Day 42 Front View Photo   Date: /   /

Day 42 Side View Photo   Date: /   /

Day 42 Back View Photo   Date: /   /

Measurements Tracker

Weight and Body Fat Percentage						
Day	Weight	Biceps	Triceps	Subscapular	Suprailiac	% BF
1						
7						
14						
21						
28						
35						
42						

Tape Measurements							
Day	**Chest/Back**	**Waist**	**Hips**	**Right Arm**	**Left Arm**	**Right Thigh**	**Left Thigh**
1							
7							
14							
21							
28							
35							
42							

Who I Am And Why You Should Listen To Me

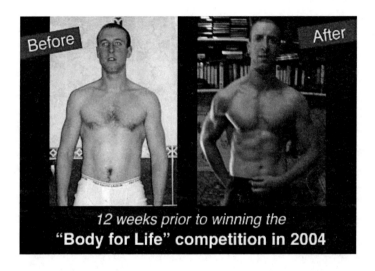

I am passionate about educating, motivating and inspiring individuals like you, athletes, entrepreneurs, teams and corporations in realising their your potential. A core foundational part of this process is regaining control over one's mind/body/health. Achieving success in this area ensures greater productivity and fast tracks results as well as leading to increased energy, focus and concentration. Importantly this also leads to you achieving success and balance in the other 3 key areas of your life - relationships, professional and wealth. As I am renowned for saying "Regaining control over your mind/body/health is the catalyst to success in all areas in life".

I have had thousands of successful clients all over the world. My focus is not just on achieving FAST results but more importantly LASTING results. I work with clients in creating balanced LIFESTYLES not temporary quick fix solutions thus creating fun, vibrant, fulfilling and successful lives.

I believe in being a role model and leader. I am a competitive Triathlete, a Body for Life Challenge Champion and Coach of Body For Life Champions 5 years running. I previously was Ireland's NSCA International Competitions Coach, shortlisted for UK Gladiators and have competed the New York and Paris Marathons among many other races. My corporate clients have included GE and Boston Scientific.

I have authored a few books as well as co-authoring many books including "Adventures in Manifesting" with Best Selling Authors such as Joe Vitale & Lorel Langemeier from "The Secret". I am currently writing a number of books.

My 20+ year career to date includes 10 Years owning and managing my own branded chain of fitness centres with over 50 staff and contractors.

I love interacting and helping my followers. So I want you to do the following :

Message me, using one of the options outlined on the Resources introduction page, and let me know your current biggest challenge.